Register Now fo
to Your

M000312769

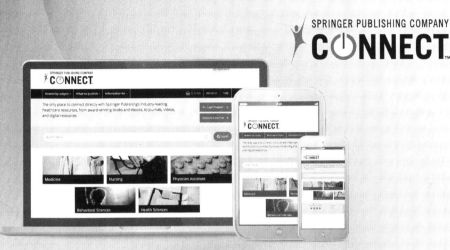

SPRINGER PUBLISHING COMPANY
C⏻NNECT™

Your print purchase of *Genetics and Genomics in Nursing,* **includes online access to the contents of your book**—increasing accessibility, portability, and searchability!

Access today at:
http://connect.springerpub.com/content/book/978-0-8261-4562-8 or scan the QR code at the right with your smartphone and enter the access code below.

R7C2J7DP

Scan here for quick access.

CS

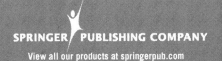

SPRINGER PUBLISHING COMPANY
View all our products at springerpub.com

Genetics and Genomics
in Nursing

Quannetta T. Edwards, PhD, MSN, MPH, FNP-BC, WHNP, AGN-BC, FAANP, is a professor in the College of Graduate Nursing at Western University of Health Sciences, Pomona, California. She has more than 44 years of experience as a registered nurse and nearly 40 years of experience as a nurse practitioner. Dr. Edwards has extensive training in the area of genetics/genomics. Her initial training began via a web-based genetics course (Genetics Education Program for Nurses) from the Cincinnati Children's Hospital, Cincinnati, Ohio. She later attended the National Institute of Nursing Research Summer Genetics Institute program at the National Institutes of Health in 2004 and completed a 2-year postdoctoral nurses' training program in clinical cancer genetics at the Department of Clinical Cancer Genetics, City of Hope, Duarte, California, from 2005 to 2007. She has given numerous local, state, and international presentations on a wide range of genetic/genomic topics and has written many peer-reviewed publications on genetics/genomics including research and review articles. Dr. Edwards has been a consultant on genetic/genomic issues for the National Institute of Nursing Research as well as other professional organizations and universities. She was an Advisory Committee member for the 2011 American Nurses Association's development of the *Essential Genetic and Genomic Competencies for Nurses With Graduate Degrees.* Dr. Edwards also provided assistance with the development of the American Nurses Credentialing Center (ANCC) guidelines and scope for Advanced Genetics Nurse Board Certification (AGN-BC). She is an editor and author of the textbook titled *Genomic Essentials for Graduate Level Nurses* (2016). Besides her work in genetics/genomics, she completed a master's degree in public health and does humanitarian missions in Africa working with people with the genetic disorder of albinism.

Ann H. Maradiegue, PhD, MSN, FNP, FAANP, is a nurse practitioner consultant. She has more than 43 years of experience as a registered nurse and 20 years of experience as a nurse practitioner. Dr. Maradiegue has extensive training in the area of genetics/genomics. Her initial training began with the National Institute of Nursing Research Summer Genetics Institute program at the National Institutes of Health in 2004. This training was followed by a 1-year intensive course in clinical cancer genetics from the Department of Clinical Cancer Genetics at the City of Hope, Duarte, California. She has given numerous local, state, and international presentations on a wide range of genetic/genomic topics and has written peer-reviewed publications on genetics/genomics including research and review articles. She has been a consultant on genetic/genomic issues for many organizations and universities and was on the 2011 American Nurses Association Consensus Panel for the development of the *Essential Genetic and Genomic Competencies for Nurses With Graduate Degrees.* She is an editor and author of the textbook titled *Genomic Essentials for Graduate Level Nurses* (2016). Dr. Maradiegue continues to work in the community with the underserved, promoting genetic access in primary care.

Genetics and Genomics in Nursing

Guidelines for Conducting a Risk Assessment

Quannetta T. Edwards, PhD, MSN, MPH, FNP-BC, WHNP, AGN-BC, FAANP

Ann H. Maradiegue, PhD, MSN, FNP, FAANP

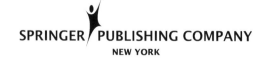

SPRINGER PUBLISHING COMPANY
NEW YORK

Springer Publishing Company, LLC
11 West 42nd Street
New York, NY 10036
www.springerpub.com

Acquisitions Editor: Joseph Morita
Compositor: Westchester Publishing Services

ISBN: 978-0-8261-4561-1
ebook ISBN: 978-0-8261-4562-8

17 18 19 20 / 5 4 3 2 1

The author and the publisher of this Work have made every effort to use sources believed to be reliable to provide information that is accurate and compatible with the standards generally accepted at the time of publication. Because medical science is continually advancing, our knowledge base continues to expand. Therefore, as new information becomes available, changes in procedures become necessary. We recommend that the reader always consult current research and specific institutional policies before performing any clinical procedure. The author and publisher shall not be liable for any special, consequential, or exemplary damages resulting, in whole or in part, from the readers' use of, or reliance on, the information contained in this book. The publisher has no responsibility for the persistence or accuracy of URLs for external or third-party Internet websites referred to in this publication and does not guarantee that any content on such websites is, or will remain, accurate or appropriate.

Library of Congress Cataloging-in-Publication Data

Names: Edwards, Quannetta T., author. | Maradiegue, Ann H., author.
Title: Genetics and genomics in nursing : guidelines for conducting a risk assessment / Quannetta T. Edwards, Ann H. Maradiegue.
Description: New York, NY : Springer Publishing Company, LLC, [2017] | Includes bibliographical references and index.
Identifiers: LCCN 2017012068 | ISBN 9780826145611 (hard copy : alk. paper) | ISBN 9780826145628 (ebook)
Subjects: | MESH: Genetic Testing—methods | Risk Assessment—methods | Genetics, Medical | Genomics | Nurses' Instruction
Classification: LCC RB155 | NLM QZ 52 | DDC 616/.042—dc23
LC record available at https://lccn.loc.gov/2017012068

Contact us to receive discount rates on bulk purchases.
We can also customize our books to meet your needs.
For more information please contact: sales@springerpub.com

Printed in the United States of America by Publishers' Graphics.

Contents

PART I. Introduction to Genetics/Genomics

PART II. Introduction to the Genomic Risk Assessment: A Step-by-Step Process

PART III. Special Populations

Contributors

Jill Fonda Allen, MS, CGC, is a board-certified genetics counselor (CGS) at the Wilson Genetics Center and the Maternal–Fetal Medicine (MFM) program in the Department of Obstetrics and Gynecology at the George Washington University Medical Center, Washington, DC. Ms. Fonda Allen received her undergraduate degree in biology from The Pennsylvania State University. She then attended Sarah Lawrence College to earn a master's degree in human genetics/genetic counseling. Ms. Fonda Allen specializes in preconception and maternal care, providing genetic counseling on prenatal screening and prenatal diagnosis. She also sees individuals and couples for genetic carrier screening, those who have a family history of a genetic condition or birth defect that may affect their children, and pregnant women taking medication or having other exposures.

Lisa M. Freese, MEd, MS, CGC, received her bachelor of science in biology and master of science in genetic counseling from the University of Pittsburgh and a master's degree in secondary education from George Washington University in Washington, DC. She is board certified in genetic counseling. After a year working in Delaware, she joined the team at the Wilson Genetics Center and the Maternal–Fetal Medicine program in the Department of Obstetrics and Gynecology at the George Washington University Medical Center, Washington, DC where she has practiced for more than 20 years. In addition to her clinical expertise, Ms. Freese has been a part of the teaching faculty at the George Washington University Medical School and is an adjunct assistant professor in the OB/GYN department.

Charles J. Macri, MD, FACOG, FACMGG, is professor of obstetrics and gynecology at the George Washington University School of Medicine and

Health Sciences, Washington, DC. He serves as the division director of Maternal–Fetal Medicine (MFM), and is associate director of the Wilson Genetics Center at George Washington University, in Washington, DC. Dr. Macri graduated from Fordham University in New York City. After receiving his medical doctorate from the Medical College of Virginia Commonwealth University, he completed an internship in obstetrics and gynecology at the Naval Medical Center in San Diego, California. Dr. Macri finished his residency in obstetrics and gynecology in San Diego and then completed fellowships in maternal–fetal medicine at the University of Southern California Los Angeles County Women's Hospital and medical genetics at the University of Southern California Children's Hospital in Los Angeles. Upon completion of his fellowship training, Dr. Macri worked at the National Naval Medical Center and the Armed Forces Institute of Pathology while also serving as a specialist in maternal–fetal medicine and medical genetics. He has worked at the George Washington University School of Medicine and Health Sciences since 2003.

Preface

The science of genetics is not a new phenomenon; rather, it dates back as early as 1865 with Gregor Johann Mendel's discovery of the basic principles of heredity as a result of certain traits found in pea plants. This discovery was significant, particularly as it related to the concepts of dominant and recessive traits (Bateson & Mendel, 1913), which play an integral role in understanding genetic disorders associated with *Mendelian inheritance*. In 1902, the condition known as *alkaptonuria* or black urine disease, an autosomal recessive disorder, was discovered because of genes associated with Mendelian inheritance (Garrod, 1902). Since that time, important discoveries in numerous single-gene inherited disorders due to autosomal dominant, autosomal recessive, X-linked dominant, X-linked recessive, mitochondrial, and, to a lesser extent, Y-linked genetic disorders have been reported. Many of these disorders are an integral part of advanced practice registered nurses' (APRNs) training/education, including that of nurse practitioner (NP) education. There are myriad single-gene disorders that expand across the life span, affecting various body systems and impacting morbidity and mortality. Some early and familiar examples of these single-gene disorders that are usually an integral part of APRN training include sickle cell disease, Huntington's disease, Marfan syndrome, Tay–Sachs disease, cystic fibrosis, hemophilia, hemochromatosis, and thalassemia, just to name a few. In fact, there are more than 24,000 autosomal, X-linked, Y-linked, and mitochondrial genes entered to date (2017) in the Online Mendelian Inheritance in Man (OMIM) database. The OMIM database is a comprehensive, authoritative online resource that is updated daily because of new discoveries and changes in genetics (Johns Hopkins University).

Today, genetics is rapidly changing as a consequence of the Human Genome Project (HGP). The HGP is a historical discovery that was completed in April 2003, enabling for the first time the complete genetic sequencing of humans that serves as a blueprint of individuals' DNA (deoxyribonucleic acid) and leading to what is now known as the *genomic era* (National Human Genome Research Institute, 2015). The genomic era is not just about rare single-gene disorders; rather, it encompasses the entire spectrum of DNA—all of the genes and the interaction and interrelationship of genes (genome) to the environment. This era has led to numerous advances in testing, diagnosis, and treatments including new medications and drug-targeted therapies, as well as social and ethical issues that have led to new policies and policy changes like the Genetic Information Nondiscrimination Act of 2008. The age of *personalized* and *precision medicine* has also been attributed to the genomic era. These types of medical advances incorporate all levels of health care, including preventive, diagnostic, and treatment transcending beyond single-gene disorders to that of complex chronic diseases.

Health and disease are significantly impacted by genetic, biological, behavioral, and environmental influences. In today's health care, integration of *risk assessment* into clinical care is of particular importance. Integration of risk assessment into clinical practice by all health care providers is vital to the early recognition of single-gene or complex (genomic) disorders so that appropriate measures can be implemented to improve health outcomes. The assessment of genetic/genomic risk is an important tool toward health promotion, prevention, and reduction of disease risk. Genetic/genomic risk assessment includes evaluation of *all* individuals regardless of age, gender, and race/ethnicity, and is a central part of personalized care. This book provides a quick and easy format to study the basic elements and steps required for risk assessment. It is geared toward APRNs, particularly NPs and midwives who provide assessment, diagnosis, and management of care in clinical settings. The text is divided into 12 chapters, with a wide range of topics to assist APRNs in the risk assessment process. These chapter topics are as follows: (1) an introduction to risk assessment including genetics/genomics core competencies for APRNs; (2) a brief overview of genetics/genomics including basic concepts; (3) patterns of inheritance; (4) an introduction to risk assessment—review of data including personal, behavioral, environmental, and family history and the assessment of the physical examination; (5) family history—using a three-generation pedigree and common pedigree nomenclature and symbols; (6) risk identification; (7) risk probability; (8) risk communication and management including consultation/referral; (9) special populations—considerations in preconception and maternal care; (10) special populations—considerations in newborn and pediatric care; (11) special populations—considerations in cancer care; and (12) a summary of the future of genetics/genomics. Each chapter includes a brief introduction to the topic, objectives, specific content related to the topic, online resources, and "Info Boxes" that are all integral to the chapter's focus. Three chapters are presented that include the risk assessment process for special populations pertaining to preconception and prenatal care, newborn and pediatric care, and cancer, specifically assessing risks for breast and colon cancer. Challenges and limitations in the genomic risk assessment are addressed, particularly as they relate to history data and pedigree interpretation. This book serves as a quick reference to use in clinical practice as well as a means to expand APRNs' knowledge, skills, and attitudes regarding genetics/genomics, genomic risk assessment, genetic conditions/disorders/diseases, and referral agencies.

References

Bateson, W., & Mendel, G. (1913). *Mendel's principles of heredity*. Cambridge, UK: Cambridge University Press.

Garrod, A. E. (1902). About alkaptonuria. *Medico-Chirurgical Transactions*, *85*, 69–78.

Johns Hopkins University. (n.d.). OMIM®—Online Mendelian Inheritance in Man®. Retrieved from http://omim.org/about

National Human Genome Research Institute. (2015). All about the Human Genome Project (HGP). Retrieved from http://www.genome.gov/10001772/all-about-the-human-genome-project-hgp

I

INTRODUCTION TO GENETICS/GENOMICS

Part I provides an overview of genetics/genomics, which is essential to the risk assessment process. In Part I, the focus is on understanding single-gene disorders. Chapter 1 describes the essential genetic and genomic competencies for nurses with graduate degrees to guide nurses in the application of their professional skills and responsibilities. Chapter 2 begins with an overview of genetics, which includes genetic sequencing, the definition of genetic mutations (including types of mutations), and the definition of single-nucleotide polymorphisms (SNPs) and their significance regarding genetics. Chapter 3 introduces patterns of inheritance with regard to Mendelian inheritance, specifically autosomal dominant, autosomal recessive, and X-linked disorders.

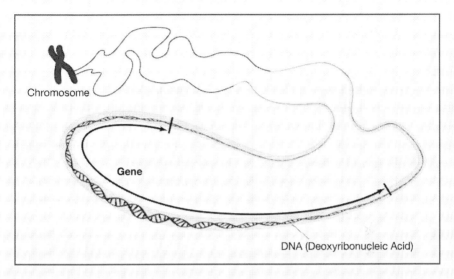

FIGURE P.I.1 A chromosome contains a single, long DNA molecule depicting a portion of a single gene.

Source: www.genome.gov/glossary/index.cfm?id=70. Courtesy of the National Human Genome Research Institute; Darryl Leja.

Objectives for Part I

1. Describe essential genetic and genomic competencies and required skills regarding the risk assessment process

2. Define common concepts used in genetics/genomics

3. Differentiate between the concepts of genetics and genomics

Additional objectives relevant to specific chapters are presented at the beginning of each chapter.

Conducting a genomic risk assessment requires that advanced practice registered nurses (APRNs) be familiar with common concepts used in genetics/genomics. Here we present some common terms that are important in the risk assessment process (see Table P.I.1).

TABLE P.I.1 Common Concepts/Terms Used in Genetics/Genomics

Concept/Term	Definition
Alleles	One of two or more versions of a gene obtained through inheritance of each parent; if two alleles are the same, they are "homozygous" for the gene; if different, they are "heterozygous" for the gene (National Human Genome Research Institute [NHGRI], 2016)
Genetics	The study of single genes and their effects (Guttmacher & Collins, 2004, p. 3; NHGRI, 2016)
Genomics	Broader term than genetics that denotes not only single genes but the entire DNA or complete genetic material including genes and their function and interaction (National Cancer Institute [NCI], n.d.)
Genotype	Individual's genetic makeup or collection of genes as determined through genetic testing
Genetic predisposition	Susceptibility or increased likelihood of developing a particular disease as a result of one's genetic makeup or genotype
Phenotype	Individual's observable characteristics (e.g., height, eye color); note the genetic contribution to these characteristics or traits indicates the genotype (NHGRI, 2016)
Pedigree	A visual genetic representation of a family tree that diagrams the inheritance of a trait or disease through multiple generations (NHGRI, 2016)

1

Risk Assessment: An Important Component of the Essential Genetic and Genomic Competencies for Nurses With Graduate Degrees

Core competencies are important to the nursing profession as they play a role in advancing mastery of nursing behaviors and skills essential to practice. Genetic/genomic-based health care is one essential core competency for today's nursing practice; it also is vital for the future of nursing. The advances in genetics/genomics are important to practice as health care moves toward significant developments in risk assessment, diagnostics, treatments, pharmacogenomics, and personalized and precision medicine that impact individuals across the life span and throughout the health and illness spectrum.

Objectives

1. Describe essential genetic and genomic competencies for nurses with graduate degrees

2. State specific skills required for advanced practice registered nurses (APRNs) regarding the risk assessment process

In September 2011, a consensus panel was established through the American Nurses Association and the International Society of Nurses in Genetics to identify essential genetic and genomic competencies for nurses trained at the graduate level as an APRN (Greco, Tinley, & Seibert, 2012). The panel included three steering committee members and 28 advisory committee and consensus panel members from various professional, state, and/or university affiliates. During this process, 38 competencies were identified and organized into eight categories that were considered the essential genetic and genomic competencies for nurses with graduate degrees. The specific title of the completed document is the *Essential Genetic and Genomic Competencies for Nurses With Graduate Degrees* (Greco et al., 2012). *Risk assessment and interpretation* is considered an essential competency of professional practice, particularly for APRN's practice, and is included in the document. The competency entails various measures for risk assessment including history-taking and assessment of risk to "identify clients with inherited predispositions to diseases as appropriate to the nurse's practice setting" (Greco et al., 2012, p. 10). Specific skills for meeting the risk assessment and interpretation competency include the following:

1. Pedigree analysis for identification of potential inherited predisposition to disease

2. Estimation of risks for Mendelian and multifactorial disorders

3. Use of family history and pedigree for targeted physical assessment

4. Interpretation of findings based on myriad data collection that includes personal and family history, physical assessment, and ancillary data (e.g., laboratory, diagnostic tests, radiology) that may indicate *suspicion* for genetic/genomic disease, disease risk, or need for referral

5. Use of referral for at-risk family members for further assessment of inherited predisposition to disease (Greco et al., 2012, p. 10)

Other important competencies of professional practice that are linked to risk assessment and interpretation include graduate nurses providing *genetic education, counseling, testing,* and *results interpretation* based on their scope of practice and clinical setting, as well as providing *consultation where appropriate;* implementing *clinical management* into client care based on assessment data and utilizing genetic referrals or other resources when needed; and ensuring *ethical, legal,* and *social issues* are considered and applied where applicable based on the assessment (Greco et al., 2012).

Conducting a genomic risk assessment entails basic *knowledge of genetics* as well as an *understanding* of the patterns of Mendelian inheritance, with knowledge of inherited/familial disorders as well as complex diseases that are a part of personal, familial, behavioral, or environmental factors. The genomic risk assessment requires *skills* to assess the multifactors that contribute to disease risk (e.g., biological, behavioral, and/or environmental)—the ability to synthesize important information, to identify red flags that may suggest disease risk or predisposition to a genetic condition, and to provide appropriate risk communication while considering ethical, legal, and social implications that may arise from genetic testing, if needed. Further, one's *attitude* regarding genetics/genomics should be one of lifelong learning for practice integration and to improve client outcomes regarding early identification of disease risk and measures to reduce adverse outcomes. Implementing a genomic risk assessment requires that APRN's knowledge and skills are kept up to date due to rapid changes and future genomic advances in testing, diagnosis, treatment, and prevention of disease. The next chapter begins with the knowledge element required for genomic risk assessment by way of a brief overview and review of genetics/genomics, which includes commonly used concepts/terms as well as patterns associated with Mendelian inheritance.

Info Box

The *Essential Genetic and Genomic Competencies for Nurses With Graduate Degrees* is an important document that describes the genetic and genomic competencies essential for nurses prepared at the graduate level, including APRNs/nurse practitioners (NPs). It includes specific competencies unique to APRNs that entail risk assessment and interpretation; genetic education; counseling, testing, and results interpretation; clinical management; and ethical, legal, and social implications.

For more information on the competencies, the reader should visit www.nursingworld.org/MainMenuCategories?Ethics Standards?Genetics-1/Essential-Genetic-and-Genomic-Com petencies-for-Nurses-With-Graduate-Degrees.pdf.

Summary

The *Essential Genetic and Genomic Competencies* for APRNs were introduced, as they are considered core competencies and skills that all APRNs should acquire in clinical and nonclinical roles. These competencies provide the framework for the practice information provided in the subsequent chapters in this text.

References

Greco, K. E., Tinley, S., & Seibert, D. (2012). *Essential genetic and genomic competencies for nurses with graduate degrees*. Silver Spring, MD: American Nurses Association and International Society of Nurses in Genetics.

Guttmacher, A. E., & Collins, F. S. (2004). Genomic medicine—A primer. In A. E. Guttmacher, F. S. Collins, & J. M. Drazen (Eds.), *Genomic medicine*. Baltimore, MD: Johns Hopkins University Press.

National Cancer Institute. (n.d.). NCI dictionary of cancer terms. Retrieved from https://www .cancer.gov/publications/dictionaries/cancer-terms?cdrid=446543

National Human Genome Research Institute. (2016, August 22). Talking glossary of genetic terms. Retrieved from https://www.genome.gov/glossary

2

Overview: Genetics/Genomics

An important part of the genomic risk assessment is having a basic knowledge and understanding of genetics, genomics, and patterns of inheritance. It is well known that genomics impacts all aspects of health and illness across the life span. It is important to know the basic elements of an individual's deoxyribonucleic acid (DNA) and how variations or alterations in the structure of one's DNA can impact health and lead to a variety of diseases, whether due to inherited or complex/multifactorial issues including the combination of genetics and environmental factors. Understanding how variation in genes, like that of a *mutation*, impacts disease is important in understanding inherited disorders like sickle cell disease, hereditary breast and colon cancer syndromes, and numerous other genetic disorders.

Objectives

1. Discuss common terms related to genetics

2. Differentiate between autosomes and sex chromosomes

3. Discuss gene sequencing and its significance in health and illness

Most individuals are born with a set of 46 normal chromosomes, obtaining 23 each from their mother and father during conception (Figure 2.1). The chromosomes are often depicted in alignment as pairs (one received

9

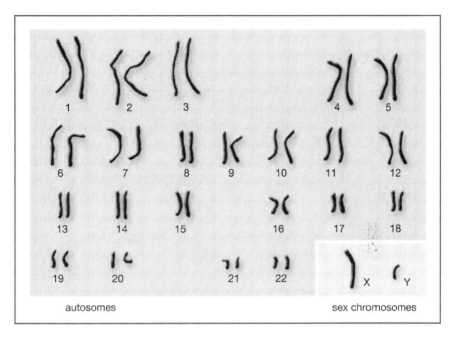

autosomes   sex chromosomes

FIGURE 2.1 Forty-six (46) human chromosomes containing 22 pairs of autosomes and one pair of sex chromosomes; this image denotes a male.

Source: U.S. National Library of Medicine.

from the mother, the other from the father) from largest to smallest, with the first 22 pairs referred to as *autosomes*; these are the same for both male and female. The last pair contains chromosomes that determine one's gender and are considered the *sex chromosomes*; if an individual has two X chromosomes, this indicates female gender; in contrast, one X and one Y chromosome indicate male gender. This alignment is depicted in a *karyotype* (Figure 2.1). The number, size, and structure of the chromosomes are important because changes in any of these qualities may result in potential problems as these chromosomes contain important genetic information. For example, individuals who have an extra chromosome 21 (e.g., 47 chromosomes), specifically three chromosomes instead of two, will have a condition known as *trisomy 21* or *Down syndrome*.

The 46 chromosomes are tightly coiled by protein substances called histones to form *nucleosomes*. These *DNA*-packaged structures are the basis of each person's hereditary information, the material of which is located in the *nucleus* of every cell of the body (Figure 2.2) with the exception of red blood cells (RBCs). Reproductive cells or gametes (e.g., egg and sperm), however, only have 23 chromosomes (not paired) for conception and normal human development.

In simplest terms, the DNA molecule contains four important chemical bases known as *adenine, guanine, cytosine,* and *thiamine,* often abbreviated or represented as *A, G, C,* and *T,* respectively, that bind together like rungs of a ladder. The two sides of the ladder are composed of alternating sugar and phosphate units, and each such unit has a nucleotide base attached to it. Hydrogen bonding between the bases holds the two strands together, forming the rungs of the ladder (Figure 2.3). One of the bases is larger, a

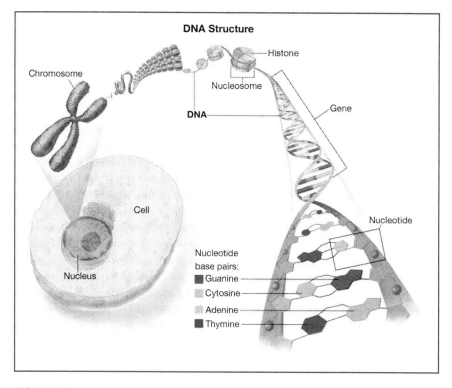

FIGURE 2.2 Structure of DNA showing a chromosome, nucleosome, histone, gene, and nucleotide base pairs: guanine, cytosine, adenine, and thymine. Also shown are a cell and its nucleus.

Source: © 2015 Terese Winslow, LLC, U.S. Govt. has certain rights. Used with permission.

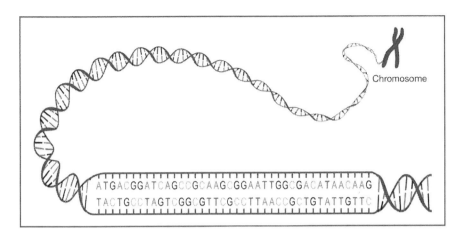

FIGURE 2.3 Example of a sequence of bases in a portion of a DNA molecule. This forms a gene that carries the instructions needed to assemble a protein.

Source: www.genome.gov/glossary/index.cfm?id=1. Courtesy of the National Human Genome Research Institute; Darryl Leja.

purine, and the other is smaller, a *pyrimidine.* The purines are adenine and guanine (A and G), and the pyrimidines are cytosine and thymine (C and T). The pyrimidine thymine (T) always pairs with the purine adenine (A) and the pyrimidine cytosine (C) always pairs with the purine guanine (G). This consistent pairing is essential when the DNA replicates itself during cell division and when decoding takes place during transcription and translation to form proteins. In the human body, the DNA consists of approximately *3 billion pairs of A, G, C, and T bases.* Alignment of these bases on the chromosome is known as a *gene*—the basic physical and functional unit of heredity. Specifically, the sequence of the A, T, C, and G makes up a gene that can vary from a few hundred to 2 million base pairs; this sequence of base pairs is *approximately 99% the same* for all people. The human body has approximately 20,000 to 25,200 genes.

Genetic sequencing of the base pairs (A, T, C, and G) is important because it forms encoded proteins that are the blueprint instructions for the structure and functioning of the human body. The genetic code obtained through the sequence of the A, T, C, and G goes through an intricate process of *transcription*—DNA copied into a single strand of messenger ribonucleic acid (mRNA; Clancy & Brown, 2008a). In the transcription process, base pairing of A with T is replaced by A pairing with U—uracil

(U) replacing thymine (T) (Figure 2.4). The base pair sequence (A, U, C, and G) of the mRNA molecule now forms a new *three-base sequence* that corresponds to a specific amino acid—this process is known as *translation* (Clancy & Brown, 2008b). The cell reads the sequence of the three bases, known as *codons*, that relates to specific amino acids or as a stop signal for further protein synthesis (Figure 2.5). There are 64 different codons, with 61 specifying amino acids. The remaining three are used as stop signals, with some trinucleotide sequence codons producing the same amino acids (Berg, Tymoczko, & Stryer, 2002). The codons are integral to producing the 21 amino acids—the building blocks of proteins that are essential for the body's structure and function and the overall process of life (Lutvo, 2009). See Figures 2.3, 2.4, and 2.5 for the depiction of transcription, translation, and codons, and Table 2.1 for the genetic codon.

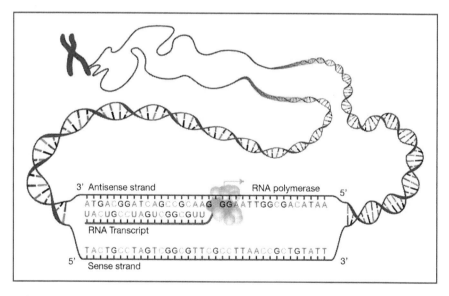

FIGURE 2.4 Transcription is the process of making a ribonucleic acid (RNA) copy of a gene sequence denoted in the RNA transcript, as depicted in the image. This copy, called a messenger RNA (mRNA) molecule, leaves the cell nucleus and enters the cytoplasm, where it directs the synthesis of the protein, which it encodes.

Source: www.genome.gov/glossary/index.cfm?id=197. Courtesy of the National Human Genome Research Institute; Darryl Leja.

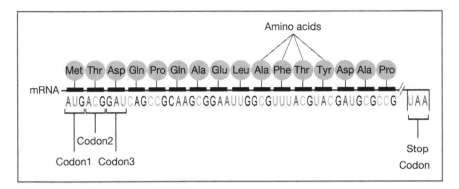

FIGURE 2.5 A messenger ribonucleic acid (mRNA) with codons that form a trinucleotide sequence of DNA or RNA that corresponds to a specific amino acid. The genetic code describes the relationship between the sequence of DNA bases (A, C, G, and T) in a gene and the corresponding protein sequence that it encodes.

Source: www.genome.gov/glossary/index.cfm?id=1. Courtesy of the National Human Genome Research Institute.

What Is the Significance of DNA Sequencing?

Some alterations in DNA sequencing based on a nucleotide(s) have the potential for change in an amino acid that can have an impact on the structure and function of the human body. The alteration, known as a *mutation,* is the basis of human diversity but can also impact health and development. *Deleterious genetic mutations* can result in a change in normal body characteristics or normal physiology. The mutation can occur in the germline (*inherited* from a parent), resulting in mutation in every cell of the body, presenting at birth and throughout life. In contrast, the mutation can be acquired spontaneously (*somatic*), due to genetic/environmental influences; this type of mutation does not present at birth, occurs in certain cells, and is not inherited (U.S. National Library of Medicine [NLM], 2016a, August 16). There are also different types of mutations. For example, some mutations may have an inherited *change in only one nucleotide* that results in a different amino acid that leads to disease. Such is the case with sickle cell anemia, where a gene mutation in chromosome 11 occurs in one segment of the gene sequence, changing from a *normal GAG sequence* to a *GTG mutation* (change in A to T). This inherited condition results in a change of the normal protein of glutamic acid to that of a

TABLE 2.1 Codons With Trinucleotide Sequences (A, C, G, U) With Corresponding Amino Acids and Start and Stop Codons

Codon	Amino Acid	Codon	Amino Acid	Codon	Amino Acid	Codon	Amino Acid
UUU	Phenylalanine	UCU	Serine	UAU	Tyrosine	UGU	Cysteine
UUC	Phenylalanine	UCC	Serine	UAC	Tyrosine	UGC	Cysteine
UUA	Leucine	UCA	Serine	UAA	STOP	UGA	STOP
UUG	Leucine	UCG	Serine	UAG	STOP	UGG	Tryptophan
CUU	Leucine	CCU	Proline	CAU	Histidine	CGU	Arginine
CUC	Leucine	CCC	Proline	CAC	Histidine	CGC	Arginine
CUA	Leucine	CCA	Proline	CAA	Glutamine	CGA	Arginine
CUG	Leucine	CCG	Proline	CAG	Glutamine	CGG	Arginine

(*continued*)

TABLE 2.1 Codons With Trinucleotide Sequences (A, C, G, U) With Corresponding Amino Acids and Start and Stop Codons (continued)

Codon	Amino Acid	Codon	Amino Acid	Codon	Amino Acid	Codon	Amino Acid
AUU	Isoleucine	ACU	Threonine	AAU	Asparagine	AGU	Serine
AUC	Isoleucine	ACC	Threonine	AAC	Asparagine	AGC	Serine
AUA	Isoleucine	ACA	Threonine	AAA	Lysine	AGA	Arginine
AUG	Methionine (START codon)	ACG	Threonine	AAG	Lysine	AGG	Arginine
GUU	Valine	GCU	Alanine	GAU	Aspartic acid	GGU	Glycine
GUC	Valine	GCC	Alanine	GAC	Aspartic acid	GGC	Glycine
GUA	Valine	GCA	Alanine	GAA	Glutamic acid	GGA	Glycine
GUG	Valine	GCG	Alanine	GAG	Glutamic acid	GGG	Glycine

Note: The amino acids are often abbreviated as follows: phenylalanine (Phe); leucine (Leu); isoleucine (Ile); valine (Val); serine (Ser); proline (Pro); threonine (Thr); alanine (Ala); tyrosine (Tyr); histidine (His); asparagine (Asn); lysine (Lys); aspartic acid (Asp); glutamic acid (Glu); cysteine (Cys); tryptophan (Trp); arginine (Arg); glycine (Gly).

mutant valine protein, resulting in abnormal hemoglobin formation and the serious disease of sickle cell anemia (Alexy et al., 2010). Mutations can be any one of the following types: a single point mutation that leads to a substitution of one amino acid for another (*missense mutation*); a change in a nucleotide that "stops" the signal for continuation of protein development (*nonsense mutation*); or an addition (*insertion*) or removal

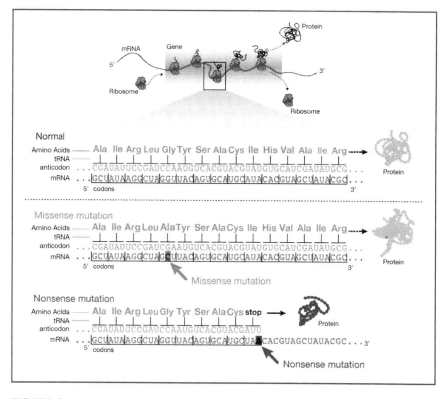

FIGURE 2.6 Example of normal DNA gene sequencing and changes that can occur due to missense mutation (protein change arginine [CGA] to alanine [GCU]) and nonsense mutation (isoleucine and rest of amino acids are stopped).

Ala, alanine; Arg, arginine; Asn, asparagine; Asp, aspartic acid; Cys, cysteine; Glu, glutamic acid; Gly, glycine; His, histidine; Ile, isoleucine; Leu, leucine; Lys, lysine; mRNA, messenger ribonucleic acid; Phe, phenylalanine; Pro, proline; Ser, serine; Thr, threonine; tRNA, transfer ribonucleic acid; Trp, tryptophan; Tyr, tyrosine; Val, valine.

Source: www.genome.gov/glossary/index.cfm?id=138. Courtesy of the National Human Genome Research Institute; Darryl Leja.

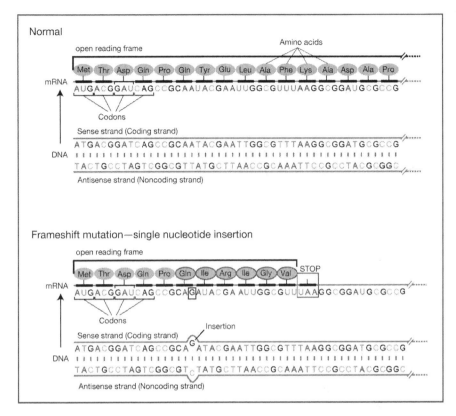

FIGURE 2.7 Example of a frameshift mutation involving the insertion or deletion of a nucleotide disrupting the reading frame of the normal three-codon sequence, leading to the entire DNA sequence following the mutation being read incorrectly.

Ala, alanine; Arg, arginine; Asp, aspartic acid; DNA, deoxyribonucleic acid; Gln, gluatamine; Glu, glutamic acid; Gly, glycine; Ile, isoleucine; Leu, leucine; Lys, lysine; mRNA, messenger ribonucleic acid; Met, methionine; Phe, phyenlalanine; Pro, proline; Thr, threonine; Tyr, tyrosine; Val, valine.

Source: www.genome.gov/glossary/index.cfm?id=68. Courtesy of the National Human Genome Research Institute; Darryl Leja.

(*deletion*) of a nucleotide base that alters the normal three-codon sequencing and thus the amino acid (*frameshift mutation*). See Figures 2.6 and 2.7 for examples of these types of mutations.

Since genes are found on chromosomes, any alteration of a chromosome—including its arrangement, assembly, or number—can also alter health and lead to structural or functional conditions or diseases in

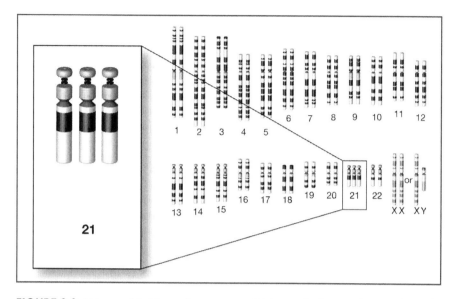

FIGURE 2.8 Trisomy 21 (three chromosome 21 instead of normal two). An individual with Down syndrome inherits all or part of an extra copy of chromosome 21. Symptoms associated with the syndrome include mental retardation, distinctive facial characteristics, and increased risk for heart defects and digestive problems, which can range from mild to severe.

Source: www.genome.gov/glossary/index.cfm?id=54. Courtesy of the National Human Genome Research Institute; Darryl Leja.

humans like Down syndrome (Figure 2.8). Chromosomal abnormalities, such as translocations, deletions, duplications, inversion of sections or ring formations, can affect genes along the chromosome and disrupt the proteins made from those genes leading to problems with growth, development, and body functions (National Human Genome Research Institute [NHGRI], 2016). Figure 2.9 is a depiction of a portion of a chromosome transferred to another (translocation).

What About Single-Nucleotide Polymorphisms (SNPs)?

Nucleotide variations do occur in humans, usually at a frequency of every 300 nucleotides, with approximately 10 million SNPs occurring in the human genome (U.S. NLM, 2016b, August 23). These SNPs are common

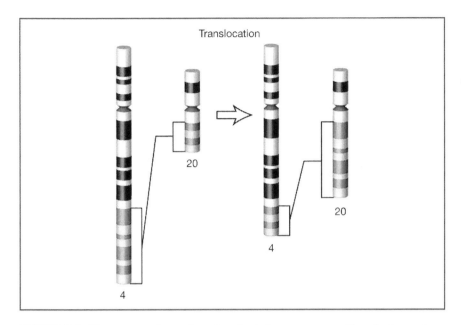

FIGURE 2.9 Chromosomal translocation depicting segments of breaks from chromosomes 4 and 20 that have reattached and translocated or changed places to the other chromosome.

Source: www.genome.gov/glossary/index.cfm?id=201. Courtesy of the National Human Genome Research Institute.

human variations with an allele frequency of at least 1% in the population (National Cancer Institute [NCI], n.d.). SNPs occur when a single nucleotide is replaced with another nucleotide. Some SNPs lead to disease, particularly if a different protein occurs that affects the structure or function of the body; however, many SNPs do not cause disease. Some SNPs have also been associated with how individuals react to drugs and other organisms (e.g., bacteria) as well as the development of disease, including possible association with chronic diseases. Thus, SNPs have a significant impact on health and illness (U.S. NLM, 2016b, August 23). A variant of uncertain significance (VUS) is often used to define a change in the genetic sequence that has occurred, which may be rare or novel; however, whether the change is associated with an increased risk of disease is unclear or unknown. Thus, pathogenicity cannot be confirmed or ruled out (National Coalition for Health Professional Education in Genetics [NCHPEG], 2013). A genetic test result with a VUS at the time of obtainment introduces a degree of uncertainty unless further findings of the significance of the change reveal disease occurrence or definite benign outcomes. In the upcoming chapters, the finding of VUS and how this finding may lead to challenges regarding risk communication and risk management are further discussed.

Info Box

Many tests to assess an individual's DNA for disease involve genetic sequencing that checks the "order" of the A, T, C, and G bases and determines if mutations exist (e.g., deleterious mutations). Sequencing of the DNA is not only an important tool to determine gene variants that can cause disease but also plays a role in screening, predicting and confirming disease, determining paternity, obtaining important data for forensics, and predicting response to therapy. *Risk assessment* may involve the need for genetic testing, which may use measures that involve genetic sequencing for those who have a personal or family history and/or physical examination for those who are suspect for an inherited disease. Advances in technology have led to *next-generation sequencing* (NGS) that provides comprehensive multiple gene sequencing for a large number of target genes based on assessment of the risk for breast cancer, colon cancer, heart disease, and a number of other disorders that may be attributed to different inherited gene disorders.

Summary

This chapter has provided a brief overview of genetics/genomics. An understanding of genetics/genomics is important when conducting a risk assessment; therefore, information beyond this book may be required based on one's prior education and experience. A list of resources is available in Table 2.2 to assist in understanding basic genetic/genomic concepts.

TABLE 2.2 Examples of Selected Online Resources for Basic Genetic/ Genomic Understanding

Online Resource	Description	Weblink
DNA From the Beginning	An animated primer of modern genetics including key basic concepts	www.dnaftb.org
GeneEd—developed by the National Library of Medicine in collaboration with the National Human Genome Research Institute	A variety of topics including cell biology, DNA, genes, and chromosomes	geneed.nlm.nih.gov
Genetics Home Reference—National Library of Medicine	Information about genetic conditions, genes, and chromosomes related to conditions	ghr.nlm.nih.gov
Your Genome—Wellcome Trust Sanger Institute	Information about DNA, genes, and genomes	www.yourgenome.org
Genetic/Genomics Competency Center	Genetic/genomics competency center with resources for classroom or practice: websites, books, articles, and other information including peer-reviewed resources	http://genomicseducation.net

References

Alexy, T., Sangkatumvong, S., Connes, P., Pais, E., Tripette, J., Barthelemy, J. C., . . . Coates, T. D. (2010). Sickle cell disease: Selected aspects of pathophysiology. *Clinical Hemorheology and Microcirculation, 44*(3), 155–166.

Berg, J. M., Tymoczko, J. L., & Stryer, L. (2002). Amino acids are encoded by groups of three bases starting from a fixed point. *Biochemistry* (5th ed., Sec. 5.5). New York, NY: W. H. Freeman. Retrieved from http://www.ncbi.nlm.nih.gov/books/NBK22358

Clancy, S., & Brown, W. (2008a). DNA transcription. *Nature Education, 1*(1), 41.

Clancy, S., & Brown, W. (2008b). Translation: DNA to mRNA to protein. *Nature Education, 1*(1), 101.

Lutvo, K. (2009). The atomic genetic code. *Journal of Computer Science & Systems Biology, 2,* 101–116.

National Cancer Institute. (n.d.). NCI dictionary of cancer terms. Retrieved from https://www .cancer.gov/publications/dictionaries/cancer-terms?cdrid=446543

National Coalition for Health Professional Education in Genetics. (2013). Variants of uncertain significance. Retrieved from http://www.nchpeg.org/microarray/what-do-other-results-mean

National Human Genome Research Institute. (2016, August 22). Talking glossary of genetic terms. Retrieved from https://www.genome.gov/glossary

U.S. National Library of Medicine. (2016a, August 16). Help me understand genetics— Mutations and health. *Genetics Home Reference* [Internet]. Retrieved from https://ghr.nlm.nih .gov/primer/mutationsanddisorders.pdf

U.S. National Library of Medicine. (2016b, August 23). Help me understand genetics—What are single nucleotide polymorphisms (SNPs)? *Genetics Home Reference* [Internet]. Retrieved from https://ghr.nlm.nih.gov/primer/genomicresearch/snp

3

Patterns of Inheritance

Patterns of inheritance refer to the way in which a trait can be passed from one generation to the next. Understanding patterns of inheritance is important to the risk assessment process. It helps clinicians to determine if the history is suspect for a single-gene disorder in the family or if there is a familial tendency for common chronic diseases such as heart disease, obesity, or diabetes. There are different ways that individuals can inherit genetic disorders, particularly single-gene disorders. Comprehending patterns of inheritance is an important part of the risk assessment process, especially for the recognition and identification of red flags that may indicate a genetic condition. This chapter discusses a brief overview of the patterns of inheritance.

Objectives

1. Differentiate between various patterns of inheritance including autosomal dominant (AD), autosomal recessive (AR), X-linked dominant, and X-linked recessive

2. Utilize appropriate online resources to assist in learning inherited genetic conditions

How Can Genetic Disorders Be Inherited?

Patterns of Inheritance—AD

AD inherited disorders are attributed to a single-gene mutation located on the autosomes or any one of the first 22 chromosomes (see Figure 2.1). Only one deleterious gene mutation located on its designated autosome is needed for disease occurrence, and this inheritance can occur at the time of conception from either the mother or father. Because of this dominance of inheritance, there is a 50% chance of transmission of the affected gene to the offspring with each pregnancy (Figure 3.1). This 50% probability often leads to multiple generations being affected in the family, depending upon the number of offspring. Examples of AD disorders include most hereditary breast cancer syndromes like hereditary breast and ovarian cancer (HBOC) due to mutations in the *BRCA* genes; Huntington's disease, Marfan syndrome, neurofibromatosis, achondroplasia, retinoblastoma, familial hypercholesterolemia, and most inherited colon cancer syndromes.

Patterns of Inheritance—AR

Like that of AD, AR disorders occur on the autosomes. Disorders that are AR require the genetic mutation to occur on *both chromosomes*, unlike AD disorders where only one chromosome with the gene mutation may lead to disease occurrence. Therefore, for an AR disorder/disease to occur, the offspring must inherit the mutation from *both the mother and father*. This requires that each parent must be at least a *carrier* of one affected chromosome with the gene mutation. Parents who are carriers of an AR disorder often will be without symptoms of the genetic disorder unless one of them has the affected disorder (e.g., both chromosomes with the gene mutation).

AR disorders are a result of Mendelian inheritance. If both parents are carriers of the genetic mutation, there is a 25%, or one in four, chance that the offspring will inherit the affected gene from each of the parents, resulting in disease. This probability of inheritance can occur with each pregnancy. There is also a 50% probability with each pregnancy that a child will be a carrier of the disorder (one normal gene and one mutated gene) and a 25% chance that the offspring is born without a gene mutation (both genes normal). Examples of recessive genetic disorders include, but are not limited to, sickle cell disease, cystic fibrosis, hemochromatosis, thalassemias

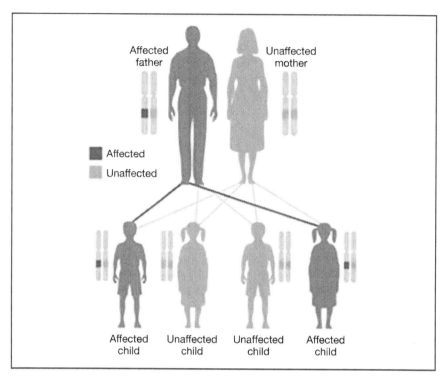

FIGURE 3.1 Autosomal dominant pattern of inheritance depicting an affected father and transmission of the gene to two of four offspring.

Source: U.S. National Library of Medicine.

(e.g., alpha thalassemia, beta thalassemia), albinism, Tay–Sachs disease, phenylketonuria (PKU), and polycystic kidney disease. In fact, most of the newborn screening (NB) tests that are mandated by public health programs are AR disorders (see Chapter 10 for information on NB screening). Figure 3.2 provides a depiction of gene transmission due to AR disorder.

Patterns of Inheritance—X-Linked Dominant

The sex chromosomes, specifically the X chromosome, are the causative factors for X-linked genetic disorders. For females, who have two X chromosomes, one affected gene mutation on the X chromosome is sufficient

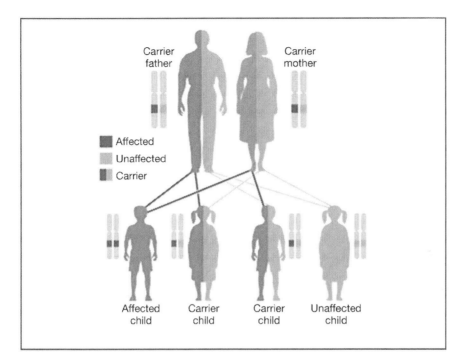

FIGURE 3.2 Autosomal recessive gene transmission with both parents being "carriers" of the gene, leading to one affected child (son) and two children who are carriers.

Source: U.S. National Library of Medicine.

for disease occurrence; because men only have one X chromosome, if the affected gene is transmitted by the mother to the son, then the male will also have the genetic disorder. In X-linked disorders, the following patterns of inheritance for disease transmission can occur with each pregnancy:

In an *affected mother*:

1. A 50%, or *one in two*, chance of transmission of the deleterious gene mutation to the female or male offspring with each pregnancy leading to the disease or condition.

2. A 50%, or *one in two*, chance that the male or female offspring will not inherit the mutated gene and will be without the disease or condition.

In an *affected father*:

1.   A 100% transmission of the disease to the female offspring occurs.

2.   No (0%) transmission to the male progeny occurs as the father only contributes the Y chromosome to male offspring.

Figure 3.3 depicts an X-linked dominant pattern of inheritance through an affected mother or father to their offspring.

There are few X-linked dominant disorders. Examples of X-linked dominant disorders include Rett syndrome, a neurodevelopmental disorder that affects primarily females (National Institute of Neurological Disorders and Strokes, 2015); hypophosphatemic rickets a disorder related to low levels of phosphate in the blood that is essential to normal bone and teeth formation (U.S. National Library of Medicine [NLM], 2017b); and incontinentia pigmenti, a disorder associated with abnormal skin changes (usually hypopigmentation) as well as numerous other

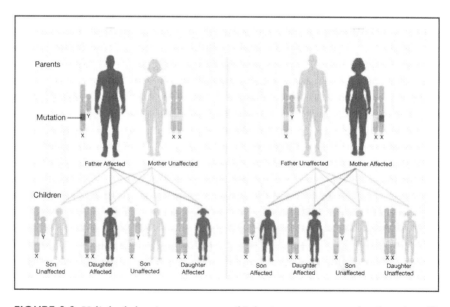

FIGURE 3.3 X-linked dominant pattern of inheritance as transmitted to the offspring from an affected father or affected mother.

Source: U.S. National Library of Medicine.

conditions including alopecia, dental abnormalities, and changes of the fingernails and toenails (U.S. NLM, 2017c).

Fragile X syndrome is another condition that results from an X-linked dominant pattern of inheritance. The prevalence of the condition is higher in males (1/4,000) compared to females (1/8,000; Jorde, Carey, & Bamshad, 2016). The syndrome is associated with intellectual, behavioral, and learning disabilities as well as numerous physical characteristics that include long face, prominent forehead and jaw, large protruding ears, connective tissue problems (e.g., hyperflexible joints; flat feet), and macroorchidism after puberty in males. Although the characteristics can be observed in both genders, males are often more severely affected by the disorder compared to females (National Fragile X Foundation, n.d.; U.S. NLM, 2017a). Figure 3.4 provides a fragile X phenotype.

Patterns of Inheritance—X-Linked Recessive

X-linked recessive disorders warrant that both genes on the female's X chromosome are affected; however, in the male, given that the offspring only has one X chromosome, a mutation on that chromosome will lead to disease. For this pattern of inheritance to cause disease, the following must occur:

1. In *female offspring*, both X chromosomes must be affected. This inheritance must occur from both parents (mother who is a carrier or affected and a father who is affected); thus, X-linked recessive disorders are rare in females.

2. In an *affected male parent* with an *unaffected female parent:*
   a. None (0%) of the male offspring will develop the disease.
   b. All daughters (100%) will be carriers but unaffected with the disease.

3. In a *female carrier* (only one X chromosome affected) with an *unaffected male:*
   a. A 50% chance that her son will be affected
   b. A 50% chance that her son will be unaffected
   c. A 50% chance that her daughter will be an unaffected carrier
   d. A 50% chance that her daughter will be unaffected and a noncarrier

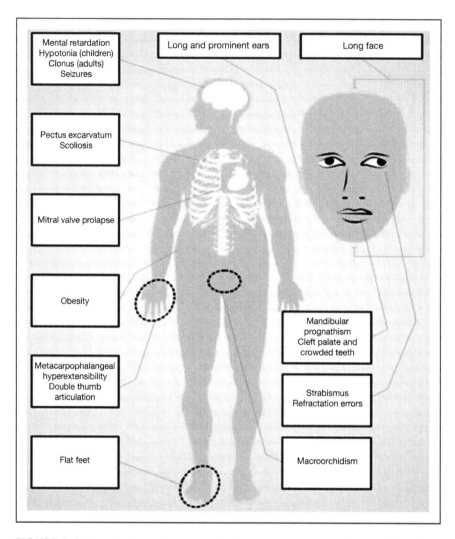

FIGURE 3.4 Description of the typical phenotypic characteristics of fragile X syndrome.

Source: Saldarriaga, Tassone, González-Teshima, Forero-Forero, Ayala-Zapata, and Hagerman (2014).

Examples of X-linked recessive disorders include hemophilia and Duchenne muscular dystrophy. Figure 3.5 displays an example of an X-linked pattern of inheritance.

Mitochondrial Inheritance

Gene mutations in the mitochondrial DNA (mtDNA) can also lead to disease. The mitochondria are located in every cell of the body (see Figure 3.6) except red blood cells; these organelles are responsible for energy generation for cell use. The mtDNA is circular and composed of only 37 genes (U.S. NLM, 2017d). Genetic mtDNA mutations are transmitted to the progeny exclusively through the mother (Sato & Sato, 2013), and *all* the children, both males and females, who inherit mtDNA will be affected with degrees of disease severity that can vary. Affected fathers never transmit the gene to the offspring (Figure 3.7). Examples of mtDNA inherited disorders from the mother include Leber hereditary optic neuropathy and Kearns–Sayre syndrome.

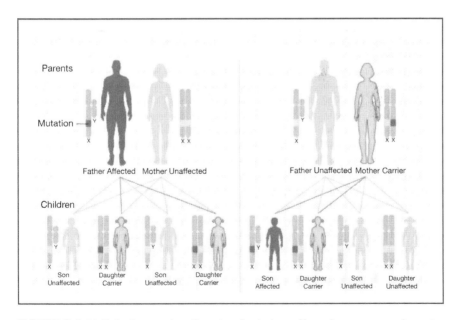

FIGURE 3.5 X-linked recessive disorder depicting affected progeny and carrier mother with transmission to offspring.

Source: U.S. National Library of Medicine.

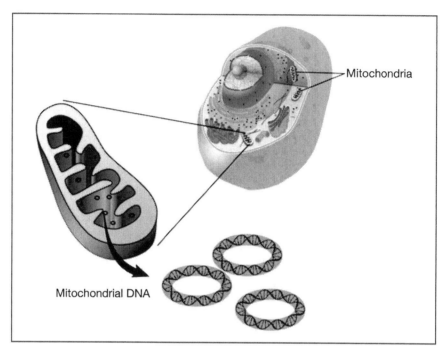

FIGURE 3.6 Mitochondrial DNA depicted as a small circular chromosome found inside mitochondria.

Source: https://www.genome.gov/glossary/index.cfm?id=129. Courtesy of the National Human Genome Research Institute; Darryl Leja.

Complex Multifactorial Disorders—Familial Impact

Most diseases are not inherited, nor do they occur due to a single-gene disorder. In fact, the majority of conditions are multifactorial, a result of genetic and environmental influences. However, since the spectrum of health and illness throughout the life span is affected by one's genome, it is important to assess the risk of chronic conditions that may be influenced by genetic, environmental, or behavioral factors. Many conditions have a *familial tendency* or a higher propensity to occur in families due to shared genes and environmental factors. Examples of complex multifactorial disorders include, but are not limited to, diabetes, most cardiovascular diseases, asthma, and obesity.

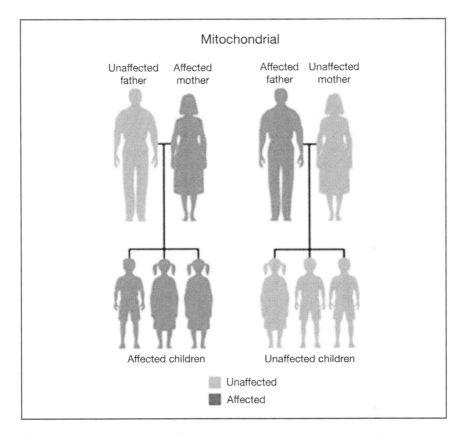

FIGURE 3.7 Mitochondrial inheritance depicting exclusive maternal transmission to the progeny regardless of the affected parent.

Source: U.S. National Library of Medicine.

Punnett Square

The Punnett square provides a way to depict the transmission of a trait based on many of the patterns of inheritance previously discussed, using a four-squared diagram, as well as knowing the genotype based on the inherited disorder. For example, if both parents are known carriers of a recessive disorder, such as sickle cell disease, the risk of each offspring having the disease, meaning they inherit both mutated alleles for sickle cell disease, can be demonstrated by a Punnett square with S = dominant normal gene and s = recessive gene for sickle cell (Figure 3.8). To illustrate, let us begin the process of drawing the Punnett square:

1. Draw a 2 × 2 square.

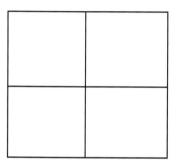

2. Assign a letter to represent the genotype. Note the genotype of *each parent* as represented by the two alleles (e.g., homozygous dominant = two copies of the dominant allele; heterozygous = two different alleles; and homozygous recessive = two recessive alleles).

3. List the genotype of each parent based on the known allele with *one parent representing columns* and the *other parent representing the rows* of the 2 × 2 square.

4. Note the contribution of each parent's alleles as noted by the inheritance of each allele to the designated area of the Punnett square.

5. Interpret and describe the findings.

Figure 3.8 is an example of a completed Punnett square of two parents; each is a sickle cell carrier, and together they have a 25% risk of a child with sickle cell disease (depicted by homozygous recessive ss genotype); a 25% probability of noncarrier and nondisease status (depicted as SS genotype/dominant homozygous), and a 50% risk of carrier (25% + 25% = 50%) status for sickle cell (depicted as Ss heterozygous).

Recognizing patterns of inheritance is integral to the risk assessment process as some conditions are inherited and have significant individual and familial implications that can impact health. The risk assessment process includes important elements such as data collection to determine disease risk, including risks for genetic disorders. The family history is an important tool in determining patterns of inheritance. Appropriate synthesis and interpretation of family history data to determine inheritance

	Paternal Genotype: S	Paternal Genotype: s
Maternal Genotype: S	SS 25%	Ss 25%
Maternal Genotype: s	Ss 25%	ss 25%

FIGURE 3.8 Punnett square with both maternal and paternal genotypes heterozygous for sickle cell (Ss) disease with the estimation of risk for sickle cell disease in the offspring for each pregnancy.

TABLE 3.1 Selected Online Resources to Enhance Learning of Patterns of Inheritance

Online Resource	Description	Weblink
Genetics Home Reference	National Library of Medicine website that contains information about genetic conditions, genes, and chromosomes related to conditions	ghr.nlm.nih.gov
GeneEd—Genetics, Education, Discovery	National Institute of Health, National Library of Medicine that provide materials on hereditary/inheritance patterns to include articles, interactive tutorials, games, videos, and other resources	geneed.nlm.nih.gov/topic_subtopic.php?tid=5
DNA Learning Center	Cold Spring Harbor Laboratory—learn about genetics: genes and inheritance; includes an animation introducing basic concepts of genetics including recessive inheritance; and Punnett squares	www.dnalc.org/resources/genescreen/inheritance.html

patterns can enable appropriate measures to be implemented for early diagnosis to prevent or reduce disease occurrence, or manage present/existing disease. The family history is particularly important in determining modes of inheritance; the use of specific tools such as the *pedigree* enables visualization of patterns to aid in identifying red flags that may denote a risk for a genetic disorder. Knowledge of patterns of inheritance is also important to communicate potential risks to other family members. Details of the family history, including the three-generation pedigree, are discussed in Chapters 4 and 5, with their application and use in clinical settings discussed throughout the book. Selected online resources to enhance learning of the patterns of inheritance are presented in Table 3.1.

Info Box

Certain genetic conditions have specific patterns of inheritance that can impact disease occurrence in the offspring:

- If one parent has an AD condition, there is a 50% probability of transmission of the affected gene to the offspring with "each pregnancy."
- If both parents are *carriers* of an AR disorder, there is a 25% probability of transmitting the affected gene to the offspring with each pregnancy.
- X-linked conditions are genetic mutations that occur on the X sex chromosome; therefore, an affected male cannot transmit the gene to his male offspring regardless if it is a dominant or recessive condition.
- Mitochondrial genetic disorders are rare, with the mutation occurring not in the cell nucleus but in the mitochondrial DNA with disease transmission to the offspring only by the mother.

Summary

This chapter has provided a brief overview of patterns of inheritance with disease examples for single gene disorders. An understanding of patterns of inheritance is important when conducting a risk assessment so that appropriate interventions can occur. A list of resources is available in Table 3.1 to assist in understanding inheritance patterns.

References

Jorde, L. B., Carey, J. C., & Bamshad, M. J. (2016). *Medical genetics* (5th ed.). Philadelphia, PA: Elsevier.

National Fragile X Foundation. (n.d.). Fragile X syndrome. Retrieved from https://fragilex.org/fragile-x/fragile-x-syndrome

National Human Genome Research Institue. (n.d.). "Talking Glossary of Genetic Terms." Retrieved from https://www.genome.gov/glossary/index.cfm?id=129

National Institute of Neurological Disorders and Stroke. (2015, July 27). Rett syndrome [Fact sheet]. Retrieved from https://www.ninds.nih.gov/disorders/rett/detail_rett.htm

Saldarriaga, W., Tassone, F., González-Teshima, L. Y., Forero-Forero, J. V., Ayala-Zapata, S., & Hagerman, R. (2014). Fragile X syndrome. *Columbia Medica, 45*(4), 190–198. Retrieved from https://openi.nlm.nih.gov/detailedresult.php?img=PMC4350386_1657-9534-cm-45-04-00190-gf01&query=fragile+X+syndrome&req=4&npos=4

Sato, M., & Sato, K. (2013). Maternal inheritance of mitochondrial DNA by diverse mechanisms to eliminate paternal mitochondrial DNA. *Biochimica et Biophysica Acta (BBA)—Molecular Cell Research, 1833*(8), 1979–1984.

U.S. National Library of Medicine. (2017a). Fragile X syndrome. *Genetics Home Reference* [Internet]. Retrieved from https://ghr.nlm.nih.gov/condition/fragile-x-syndrome

U.S. National Library of Medicine. (2017b). Hereditary hypophosphatemic rickets. *Genetics Home Reference* [Internet]. Retrieved from https://ghr.nlm.nih.gov/condition/hereditary-hypophosphatemic-rickets

U.S. National Library of Medicine. (2017c). Incontinentia pigmenti. *Genetics Home Reference* [Internet]. Retrieved from https://ghr.nlm.nih.gov/condition/incontinentia-pigmenti#inheritance

U.S. National Library of Medicine. (2017d). Mitochondrial DNA. *Genetics Home Reference* [Internet]. Retrieved from https://ghr.nlm.nih.gov/mitochondrial-dna#sourcesforpage

II

INTRODUCTION TO THE GENOMIC RISK ASSESSMENT: A STEP-BY-STEP PROCESS

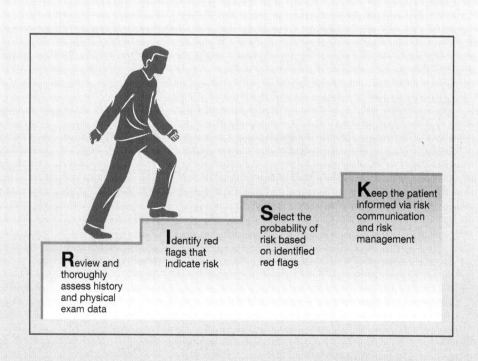

Review and thoroughly assess history and physical exam data

Identify red flags that indicate risk

Select the probability of risk based on identified red flags

Keep the patient informed via risk communication and risk management

Recognizing inheritance patterns to determine disease causation, susceptibility, or future disease prediction warrants an in-depth risk assessment that includes a thorough personal and family history, physical examination, and genetic testing, if applicable. Assessment of disease risk is important to determine not only genetic but also complex disease risks. Risk assessment is a *process* that can aid in:

- Early diagnosis and treatment to improve outcomes
- Implementation of chemoprevention to reduce risk of future disease occurrence
- Prevention of disease through lifestyle/behavioral modifications
- Implementation of enhanced surveillance for early diagnosis
- Risk-reduction measures (e.g., surgery) to lower or eliminate disease incidence
- Determination for genetic testing
- Serving as a benchmark for current and future health status

Objectives for Part II

1. State the basic components of the genomic risk assessment

2. Discuss the benefits of conducting a genomic risk assessment

Disease occurrence can result from a myriad of factors, including conditions caused by single-gene mutations that lead to hereditary disorders or noninherited complex conditions involving multifactorial genetic, environmental, or behavioral factors. An in-depth assessment to determine disease *risk* is imperative in either case to prevent or reduce disease occurrence or counter disease progression via diagnosis. This requires knowledge and *risk assessment* skills to ensure adequate data collection methods are implemented to *identify* factors that impact disease risk, to determine *risk probability* based on the identified factors, and to appropriately deliver *risk communication* and *risk management* to clients based on their risk.

Risk assessment is an ongoing process—not a one-time event—that entails an initial thorough assessment to determine risk and continues with each patient visit to update information regarding change that may indicate "new" risks that were not identified on prior visits. The steps of the process are as follows: (a) *review* of data obtained from a thorough personal and family history including assessment of laboratory and ancillary data as well as evaluation of pertinent physical examination data; (b) *identification* of red flags based on data collection and assessment that indicates the potential for genetic or familial risk; (c) *selection* of risk probability through use of family history, genetic tests, or evidence-based risk probability tools to determine the likelihood of disease occurrence (population, moderate, or high risk); and (d) *keeping* the patient informed through risk communication while also implementing risk management strategies that are evidence based, culturally appropriate, and involve shared decision making. Chapters 4 to 8 describe each of these elements via a step-by-step risk assessment process.

Info Box

The acronym *RISK* can be a useful tool in remembering the steps in the risk assessment process.

- *Review* and thoroughly assess collected data of personal and family history and any pertinent ancillary or laboratory information as well as data obtained from the physical exam.
- *Identify* data to determine elements of risk—are there red flags?
- *Select* the appropriate probability for risk occurrence—is the patient at population, moderate, or high risk for disease occurrence?
- *Keep* the patient informed through risk communication while informing him or her of strategies to manage the risk.

4

Step 1.a: Review Collected Data— Personal, Ancillary, Laboratory, and Physical Examination

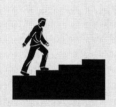

Step 1 of the genetic/genomic risk assessment process requires data collection through history-taking, physical examination, and review and interpretation of additional data (e.g., radiology, laboratory), if applicable. Data collection is an ongoing process that begins at the first clinic visit and then is updated through subsequent health provider and patient encounters. The personal history is used in conjunction with the family history as the major sources of risk assessment. An accurate in-depth assessment integrated with the physical exam provides a powerful tool for determining risk and preventing, diagnosing, and/or managing disease risk or disease occurrence. For the remainder of the book, we refer to the assessment process as the *genomic risk assessment*.

Objectives

1. Describe Step 1.a of the genetic/genomic risk assessment

2. Discuss how the physical examination may aid in identifying certain genetic conditions

Advanced practice registered nurses (APRNs) learn early in their nursing career to take an in-depth personal, family, social, and environmental history—including collection of behavioral and ancillary data—as part of the assessment process. The assessment is a systematic, deliberative, and interactive process based on data collection, validation, analysis, and synthesis for making decisions about the health status of individuals, families, and/or communities (Benner, Hughes, & Stuphen, 2008; Bickley & Szilagyi, 2013). The need for an in-depth assessment is equally important in the genomic risk assessment process. In the genomic risk assessment, the process is important for early recognition of patterns of inheritance or identification of elements in the history that may denote a present genetic disorder or a genetic predisposition for a disease. The genomic risk assessment has implications for clinical practice and risk management with regard to early diagnosis that can be of prophylactic value, more efficacious treatment for disease, and determination of the need for genetic testing for disease diagnosis and prognosis, as well as the need for monitoring disease progress. The genomic risk assessment may also provide information of *familial risks* or conditions that may occur in multiple family members, which, although not due to a single-gene disorder, may be important in management of care to reduce individual disease risk through behavioral change, chemoprevention, or enhanced surveillance for early diagnosis.

Personal History

A detailed personal history assessment must be conducted to determine genomic risk for disease occurrence. Essential information includes the following: (a) race/ethnicity; (b) ancestry of origin if known; (c) current age; (d) detailed medical and surgical history with age of disease onset and/or date of surgery; (e) present and past medications including over-the-counter (OTC) meds; (f) significant therapies; (g) history of genetic testing including type, dates, and findings; and (h) complete gynecological/reproductive and obstetrical history. Because the genomic risk assessment may involve issues related to cancer, a personal history of cancer should be obtained, if applicable, that includes the age of onset of cancer, type of cancer, pathology reports, exposure to carcinogens, reproductive history, hormone or oral contraceptive use, and surgical history including specific reason for surgery (e.g., hysterectomy for fibroids vs. cancer). Any history of chemoprevention and/or risk-reducing surgery (e.g., total abdominal hysterectomy and salpingo-oophorectomy due to a confirmed history of Lynch syndrome) should also be part of the personal history (National Comprehensive Cancer Network [NCCN], 2016). These same principles apply to all disorders dependent upon the disease/s noted in families; the data required may differ according to the family disease predisposition (e.g., heart disease and EKG; mental illness and psychiatric evaluation). Because many genetic disorders are syndromic—that is, they have more than one identifying feature, symptom, or disease associated with the disorder—it is critical that all personal data collected are reviewed and synthesized for patterns to aid in interpretation of potential genetic conditions and the determination of need to counsel or refer the patient for possible genetic testing.

Behavioral data like sexual history, smoking, and illegal drug and alcohol use should also be included in the personal history as certain exposures can impact the risk of many diseases and knowledge of behavioral data can aid in diagnosis or exaggerate certain known genetic, familial, or chronic conditions (e.g., nicotine use and cardiovascular diseases). Environmental factors like radiation exposure may increase the risk for certain conditions, particularly some cancers. Ancillary data such as laboratory, radiology, and other screening or diagnostic tests should be included in the history, noting the dates of testing and specific results as these data can provide crucial information regarding genetic disorders and genetic predisposition. For instance, the record of an individual with a history of colon polyps identified via a colonoscopy should include the type and number of polyps as a certain type and number of polyps can be suspect for inherited colon cancer syndromes (see Chapter 11 on cancer risk assessment). Similarly, certain types of breast cancer or a history of *bilaterality* (e.g., *synchronous* defined as a history of two [or more] breast cancers identified at the same time or within 6 months after the first, and is considered a "new" breast cancer and not metastatic; or *metachronous contralateral* defined as a "new" breast cancer diagnosed more than 6 months following the first cancer in the opposite breast) may be red flags that are suspect for inherited breast cancer syndromes, particularly when an early age of onset and/or family history of the disease are also present (Padmanabhan, Subramanyan, & Radhakrishna, 2015; Varsha, Manveen, Amar, & Anju, 2016). Extreme or unusual laboratory findings may also indicate a genetic disorder. For instance, familial hypercholesterolemia, an autosomal dominant (AD) genetic disorder, is associated with elevated low-density lipoprotein (LDL) levels (190 mg/dL in adults). A number of physical characteristics may also be observed in the condition (e.g., tendon xanthomas, corneal arcus younger than age 45 years; Youngblom, Pariani, & Knowles, 2016). Individuals with familial hypercholesterolemia are at risk for early age onset of death due to cardiac disease. Assessment of any prior genetic testing including the type/name of the test and test results should also be obtained from the personal history, as well as inquiry for any known genetic mutation in the family.

Physical Examination

The personal history should be followed by a *focused physical exam* based on the collected individual history as well as other data (e.g., family history, ancillary data). The physical exam provides objective information that can complement the personal and family history, aiding in diagnosis or need for further evaluation or testing (e.g., genetic testing). Examination includes observation for dysmorphology, anomalies, or other characteristics that may be suspect for an inherited disorder. The exam also provides crucial information that may be the basis for a diagnosis of genetic disease or genetic predisposition. A focused breast exam for individuals at risk for

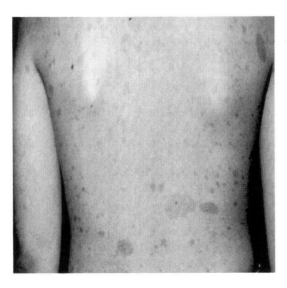

FIGURE 4.1 Café au lait spots.

Source: From Khalil, Afif, Elkacemi, Benoulaid, Kebdani, and Benjaafar. (2015).

breast cancer, for instance, should include a thorough breast exam as well as a dermatologic and oral mucosa exam, head circumference exam, and thyroid exam as these body sites may denote abnormalities that are suspect for certain hereditary breast cancer syndromes like Cowden syndrome (National Cancer Institute [NCI], 2016, July 28; NCCN, 2016). Multiple café au lait spots (Figure 4.1) may be an indicator of a genetic disorder known as neurofibromatosis type 1, particularly when these characteristics are found with other features (e.g., Lisch nodules, neurofibromas; Friedman, 1998/2014). Another genetic disorder known as Peutz–Jeghers syndrome may also manifest with mucocutaneous macules during childhood on the mouth, eyes, nostrils, perianal area, buccal mucosa, or fingers (McGarrity, Amos, & Baker, 2001/2016). These physical characteristics with other features may be suspect for the syndrome. Peutz–Jeghers syndrome is an AD genetic disorder associated with intestinal hamartomatous polyps and numerous cancers and other conditions due to mutations in the *STK11/LKB1* gene (Figure 4.2). More information on this syndrome is presented in Chapter 11.

The genomic personal assessment entails not only data review of the individual's medical, surgical, behavioral, and ancillary histories but also warrants a focused detailed physical exam. During the risk assessment process, all of the information is synthesized in order to help the provider identify risk elements that are potential red flags, quantify or qualify potential risk for specific diseases (e.g., population, moderate, high risk), and, when applicable, establish communication for prevention, diagnosis,

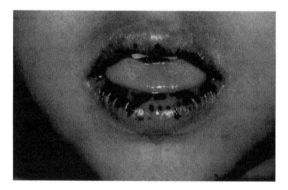

FIGURE 4.2 Peutz–Jeghers syndrome with black spots localized in the perioral area.

Source: From Gondak, da Silva-Jorge, Jorge, Lopes, and Vargas (2012).

or management of current health status. Risk assessment can also be tailored to the individual to improve health outcomes by identifying modifiable risk factors, arranging appropriate referrals, and providing behavioral and medical interventions (Goetzel et al., 2011). It is important to be knowledgeable of genetic disorders and any associated characteristics or

TABLE 4.1 Examples of Online Resources for Genetic Conditions

Online Resource	Description	Weblink
Genetics Home Reference—Health Conditions	National Library of Medicine website that contains information about signs and symptoms, frequency, genetic cause, and inheritance patterns of various conditions, diseases, and syndromes	ghr.nlm. nih.gov/ condition
Online Mendelian Inheritance in Man (OMIM)	Comprehensive authoritative compendium of human genes and genetic phenotypes authored and edited by the McKusick-Nathans Institute of Genetic Medicine, Johns Hopkins University School of Medicine, under direction of Dr. Ada Hamosh	www.ncbi.nlm.nih.gov/ omim
National Human Genome Research Institute—Specific Genetic Disorders	List of specific genetic disorders	www.genome.gov/ 10001204/specific -genetic-disorders
Cancer Genetics Risk Assessment and Counseling (PDQ®)- Health Professional Version	National Cancer Institute's summary of current approaches to assessing and counseling individuals regarding an inherited susceptibility to cancer	www.cancer.gov/about -cancer/causes -prevention/genetics/ risk-assessment-pdq

> **Info Box**
>
> - The personal history is a *process* and a crucial part of the genomic risk assessment that should be taken at the initial visit and reviewed and updated where applicable on subsequent visits.
> - Knowledge of the characteristics and physical features of a genetic condition is crucial to the genomic risk assessment, particularly when conducting a history and physical examination.

other conditions that may be related to the disorder so that counseling for genetic testing can be conducted. Although there are numerous genetic disorders, Table 4.1 provides some examples of selected resources on genetic conditions.

Summary

This chapter introduces the risk-assessment process. The process is an important part of identifying individuals who may be at risk for inherited, familial, multi-factorial, or behavioral disorders. The first step of the risk-assessment process is a thorough review of personal and family history as well as evaluation of physical findings, laboratory data, and other ancillary data if available. In the next chapter, we further expand this review process with a discussion of the importance of conducting and reviewing the family history particularly that of a three-generation pedigree.

References

Benner, P., Hughes, R., & Stuphen, M. (2008). Clinical reasoning, decision making, and action: Thinking critically and clinically. In R. Hughes (Ed.), *Patient safety and quality: An evidence based handbook for nurses* (Chap. 6). Rockville, MD: Agency for Healthcare Research and Quality. Retrieved from http://www.ncbi.nlm.nih.gov/books/NBK2643

Bickley, L. S., & Szilagyi, P. (Eds.). (2013). *Bates' guide to physical assessment and history taking. Foundations in health assessment* (11th ed., pp. 3–96). Philadelphia, PA: Lippincott Williams & Wilkins.

Friedman, J. M. (1998 [updated 2014, September 4]). Neurofibromatosis 1. In R. A. Pagon, M. P. Adam, H. H. Ardinger, S. E. Wallace, A. Amemiya, L. J. H. Bean, . . . K. Stevens (Eds.), *GeneReviews®* [Internet]. Seattle: University of Washington. Retrieved from https://www.ncbi .nlm.nih.gov/books/NBK1109

Goetzel, R. Z., Staley, P., Ogden, L., Stange, P., Fox, J., Spangler, J., . . . Taylor, M. V. (2011). A framework for patient-centered health risk assessments—Providing health promotion and disease prevention services to Medicare beneficiaries. Retrieved from http://www.cdc.gov/policy/ hst/hra/frameworkforhra.pdf

Gondak, R. O., da Silva-Jorge, R., Jorge, J., Lopes, M. A., & Vargas, P. A. (2012). Oral pigmented lesions: Clinicopathologic features and review of the literature. *Medicina Oral, Patologia Oral y Cirugia Bucal, 17*(6). Retrieved from https://openi.nlm.nih.gov/detailedresult .php?img=PMC3505710_medoral-17-e919-g003&req=4

Khalil, J., Afif, M., Elkacemi, H., Benoulaid, M., Kebdani, T., & Benjaafar, N. (2015). Breast cancer associated with neurofibromatosis type 1: A case series and review of the literature. *Journal of Medical Case Reports, 9*(61). Retrieved from https://www.ncbi.nlm.nih.gov/pmc/ articles/PMC4372231

McGarrity, T. J., Amos, C. I., & Baker, M. J. (2001 [updated 2016, July 14]). Peutz-Jeghers syndrome. In R. A. Pagon, M. P. Adam, H. H. Ardinger, S. E. Wallace, A. Amemiya, L. J. H. Bean, . . . K. Stephens (Eds.), *GeneReviews®* [Internet]. Seattle: University of Washington. Retrieved from https://www.ncbi.nlm.nih.gov/books/NBK1266

National Cancer Institute. (2016, May 11). Cancer genetics risk assessment and counseling (PDQ®)—Health professional version. Retrieved from https://www.cancer.gov/about-cancer/ causes-prevention/genetics/risk-assessment-pdq#link/_336_toc

National Comprehensive Cancer Network. (2016). Genetic/familial high-risk assessment: Breast and ovarian. Retrieved from https://www.nccn.org/professionals/physician_gls/pdf/ genetics_screening.pdf

Padmanabhan, N., Subramanyan, A., & Radhakrishna, S. (2015). Synchronous bilateral breast cancers. *Journal of Clinical and Diagnostic Research, 9*(9), XC05–XC08. doi:10.7860/ JCDR/2015/14880.6511

Varsha, D., Manveen, K., Amar, B., & Anju, B. (2016). Synchronous and metachronous bilateral breast malignancies: Report of two cases and literature review. *Journal of Gynecologic Surgery, 32*(2), 136–138.

Youngblom, E., Pariani, M., & Knowles, J. W. (2016). Familial hypercholesterolemia. In R. A. Pagon, M. P. Adam, H. H. Ardinger, S. E. Wallace; A. Amemiya, L. J. H. Bean, . . . K. Stephens (Eds.), *GeneReviews®*. Seattle: University of Washington. Retrieved from https:// www.ncbi.nlm.nih.gov/books/NBK174884

5

Step 1.b: Review Collected Data—Family History and the Use and Interpretation of the Pedigree

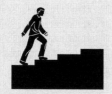

The family history is a continuation of Step 1 of data collection for the genomic risk assessment. Family history represents the health and disease conditions experienced by family members over the course of their lives. It is the family tree. The use of a pedigree to capture the family history provides a visualization of the maternal and paternal lineages of multiple generations that can provide an excellent way to observe relationships and patterns that can be suspect or diagnostic of inherited disorders and familial diseases associated with complex chronic disorders or shared environmental issues. In fact, the family history is considered by some as the *first genetic test*.

Objectives

1. Discuss common terms used in constructing a pedigree

2. Describe basic elements of the pedigree

3. Discuss the three-generation pedigree and the significance to health and illness

4. Conduct a family history using a three-generation pedigree

The family history is vital to the genomic risk assessment. Family history plays a significant role in health care, and with the evolution of medical genomics it is believed that family history contributes to the advancement of personalized health care (Wilson et al., 2012). When used with the personal history, it can (a) inform diagnosis; (b) promote risk assessment to estimate an individual's risk of developing a specific condition through risk stratification (e.g., population/average risk, moderate risk, or high risk); (c) provide a means for the prevention, diagnosis, and management of disease, with the primary emphasis on prevention; and (d) establish rapport through risk communication, allowing better health-related decision making regarding disease risk and management of care (National Coalition for Health Professional Education in Genetics [NCHPEG], 2016).

One of the most important risk assessment tools is the family history in the form of a *three-generation pedigree*. A positive family history is associated with a higher risk of a disorder when multiple family members who are first- and second-degree relatives are affected with a disease and/or the disease occurs at a younger age than normally seen in the general population. The family history is representative of the family's shared genes, environment, and behaviors (Wilson et al., 2012). Families with positive histories for frequently occurring disorders such as diabetes or heart disease have a two- to fivefold greater relative risk for disease occurrence than the general population (Reid & Emory, 2006). Advanced practice registered nurses (APRNs) can use the three-generation pedigree to offer important diagnostic and screening interventions appropriate for the identified disorder as well as preventive measures to reduce or prevent disease occurrence.

The types of family assessment include *comprehensive* and *targeted* histories (NCHPEG, 2016). The comprehensive family history is an in-depth assessment of major medical concerns, chronic medical conditions, hospitalization, surgeries, birth defects, and intellectual disabilities including mental retardation, learning disabilities, or developmental delays that may occur in the family. In contrast, a targeted family history directs questions related to a particular disorder (e.g., cancer, heart disease, hearing loss), either concerning a positive family history of disorders in relatives or an individual's history of present illness (NCHPEG, 2016). In the clinical setting, the level of suspicion based on personal history or other data influences the collection and application of the family history. Using information gleaned from the family history and coupled with the personal history and ancillary data, provisions can be made for patients based on their disease risk. For example, individuals with multiple family members who have a disorder (e.g., first- and second-degree members with breast cancer) may indicate the need for further evaluation to determine if the patient has a predisposition to breast cancer based on an inherited genetic disorder (e.g., hereditary breast and ovarian cancer [HBOC] due to mutation in a *BRCA* gene or other inherited breast cancer genes). Individuals with a genetic mutation for most breast cancer syndromes would be considered at high risk for the disease. In contrast, a patient whose personal and family history is unremarkable or uneventful may be at average or population risk for breast cancer. The family history with other data (personal history) aids in determination of a probability for disease risk; implementation of screening measures for early detection of disease, behavioral modifications (e.g., smoking cessation), or chemoprevention to reduce risk (e.g., aspirin therapy and cardiovascular disease); or consideration of risk-reducing surgery to further reduce risk.

Family history is an important tool for prevention and disease recognition that can be applied to various settings. Collection of family history data should be a continuous process that is evaluated and updated during each client contact (Bennett, 2010).

Three-Generation Pedigree

A basic pedigree consists of a minimum of three generations: first-degree relatives (e.g., parents, children, siblings), second-degree relatives (half siblings, grandparents, aunts and uncles, grandchildren), and third-degree relatives (cousins, great-grandparents, great-grandchildren). The *consultand* is the person with the appointment, seeking health care or genomic health information. This person is identified on the pedigree with an arrow. The consultand can be healthy or a person with a medical condition. The *proband* is the affected individual who brings the family to medical attention and may not be present during the appointment with the consultand. An individual can assume both roles, that of the consultand and the proband. The three-generation pedigree provides a graphic picture of how family members are biologically related to each other, from one generation to the next. Generally, the pedigree is collected face to face prior to the physical

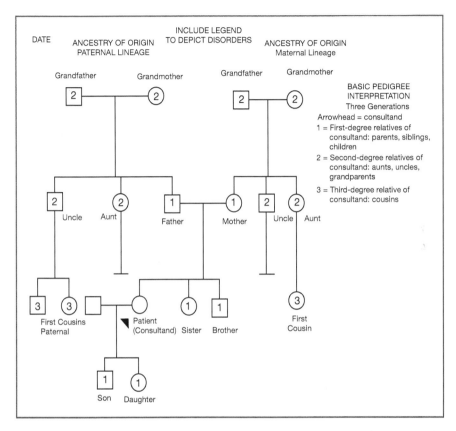

FIGURE 5.1 Basic pedigree demonstrating three generations with first-, second-, and third-degree relatives.

exam. Figures 5.1 and 5.2 are examples of family pedigrees depicting members of multiple generations for both the maternal and paternal lineages. The figures include placement of members pertaining to the first, second, and third generation in the family as well as their relationship lines, and whether the member is alive or deceased. This forms the basic structure of the therapy. Additional data such as ancestry of origin and specific information regarding medical or surgical history; prior genetic testing, if applicable, with results; and other pertinent data are needed. An inclusion of a legend or key is a part of the pedigree as it pertains to specific medical or disease history.

Due to the amount of information required, many providers are using forms to have the patient document detailed information prior to the

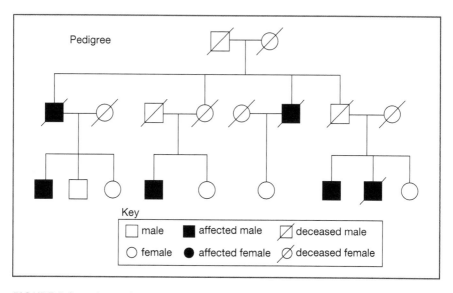

FIGURE 5.2 Pedigree from a chart depicting relationships with legend.

Source: http://www.accessexcellence.org/RC/VL/GG/pedigree.html. Courtesy of the National Human Genome Institute.

office visit. This method allows the patient additional time to inquire about previously unknown family history and procure documents, if needed (e.g., death certificates), as well as allows the health care provider time to review the information prior to the patient's appointment if the family history data are sent prior to the patient visit. In addition, if administrative services are provided, having the family history data prior to the appointment can allow time for preparation of the information in a pedigree format.

There are numerous symbols that are used to make a family pedigree. Standardized nomenclature and symbols for pedigree construction are noted in Figure 5.3. This figure also provides information on social and legal relationships (e.g., adoption, divorce), deaths, pregnancy termination, and use of assistive reproductive technologies. Each family member within the pedigree is recorded using appropriate symbols—a square (male) or a circle (female)—that are connected to each other. A pregnancy is represented as a diamond with a *P* inside. A diamond can also be used when it is not important to specify gender or the information is unknown, noted by placing an *n* inside. The diamond can also be used for a transgendered person or persons with congenital disorders of sexual development (chromosomal, gonadal, or anatomic). Specific information regarding gender, if known

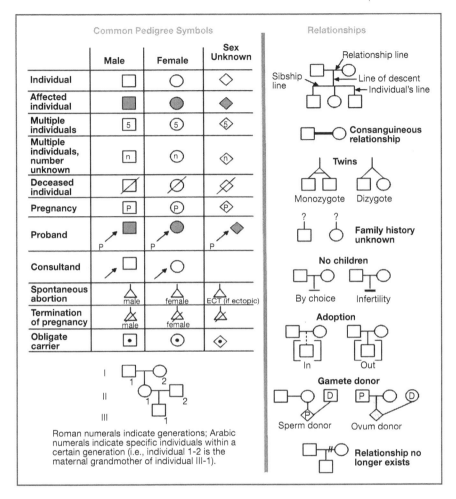

FIGURE 5.3 Examples of commonly used standard pedigree symbols.

ECT, electroconvulsive therapy.

Source: Bennett (1999). Reprinted with permission from John Wiley & Sons.

(e.g., chromosomal number), is placed below the diamond symbol; for example, 46XY indicating a male with a normal number of chromosomes. The various pedigree symbols related to pregnancy, spontaneous abortion, termination of pregnancy, and infertility are shown in Figure 5.3.

A relationship line is a horizontal line between two partners. A slash or break in that line indicates separation or divorce. A consanguineous couple (defined as a "blood relative" or having the same ancestry or descent—e.g., cousins marrying each other) should be connected by a double relationship line. The sibship (siblings) line is a horizontal line that connects brothers and sisters. The difference between sibship and partner relationship lines is that each sibling has a vertical individual line attached to the horizontal line above the individual's symbol. The line of descent is a vertical bridge connecting the horizontal sibship line to the horizontal relationship line (Bennett, 2010). It is important to record the partners of the siblings if they have a significant medical history in their offspring (e.g., autosomal recessive [AR] disorder) or if there is a family history of an identified medical condition (e.g., diabetes). Each generation should be on the same horizontal plane; for example, an individual's siblings and cousins should be on the same horizontal axis. Generally, each generation is defined by a roman numeral. First names or initials are generally recorded by the symbol for each individual to meet privacy standards. It is important to note adoption as someone who is *adopted in* (nonbiological relationship) from someone who is *adopted out* (a biological relative). If the person is adopted by an individual or a couple, a dotted line is used to indicate a nonbiological relationship, as noted in Figure 5.3. It is not uncommon for a family member to adopt a relative; for example, a sibling adopts his or her niece or nephew (adopted out).

Documenting who is affected (with a disease) and who is unaffected (without a disease) is crucial for risk analysis of the pedigree. Pedigree symbols should be shaded only for affected individuals. Different shading can be used to identify separate diseases on the pedigree. For example, when documenting a family history of multiple types of cancer, shading in the various quadrants of each square (male) and each circle (female) is a way to symbolize different types of cancer within the family. A simple way to document that an individual is disease free is to note *alive and well* under each healthy individual on the pedigree. Information about the unaffected members of the family is important. For example, if a 50-year-old woman is recently diagnosed with breast cancer but her five older sisters are cancer free, you are more likely to suspect a sporadic occurrence rather than an autosomal dominant (AD) disorder for breast cancer, especially if the remaining family history on both lineages does not represent a history suspect for an inherited breast cancer syndrome.

Race/ethnicity is also important to record because certain diseases have been identified within ethnic groups, and the sensitivity of genetic tests depends on the correct ethnic information. For example, sickle cell trait is carried in one out of 13 African American children, and one out of every

365 African American babies is born with sickle cell disease (National Heart, Lung, and Blood Institute, 2016). Sometimes little information is known about the family history. Placing a question mark above the pedigree symbol shows that you inquired about the person's medical history and the information is unknown. Some general guidelines for drawing a pedigree are provided in Table 5.1. (*Note:* When incorporating information into a pedigree format, use abbreviations sparingly to record disorders in the family and define them in a key or legend that is part of the document depicted in Figures 5.4, 5.5, and 5.6.)

TABLE 5.1 General Guidelines for Drawing a Three-Generation Pedigree

General Guidelines

- Male partners are to the left of female partners.
- Draw siblings in order from oldest to youngest, with the oldest on the left and the youngest on the right.
- For multiple disorders/diseases, use quadrants or different shading (solid, cross-hatching) to indicate each disease.
- It is just as important to record information on unaffected relatives as affected relatives.

Information That Must Be Included in a Pedigree

- First name or initials of relatives (limit identifying information to be compliant with Health Insurance Portability and Accountability Act (HIPAA) guidelines)
- Affected status (e.g., who in the family has the disease) for each individual
- Age of all family members, or age at death (do not submit a full birth date at this time to be compliant with HIPAA guidelines)
- Whether individuals are living or deceased
- Cause of death, if known, which should be indicated below the symbol
- The disease or disorder the individual has, along with the age of onset below the symbol
- Key to shading of symbols
- Adoption status if applicable
- Consanguinity (e.g., parents are related)
- At the top, note the ethnicity of each grandparent (e.g., French, African American)
- Date pedigree obtained

Source: Bennett, French, Resta, and Doyle (2008).

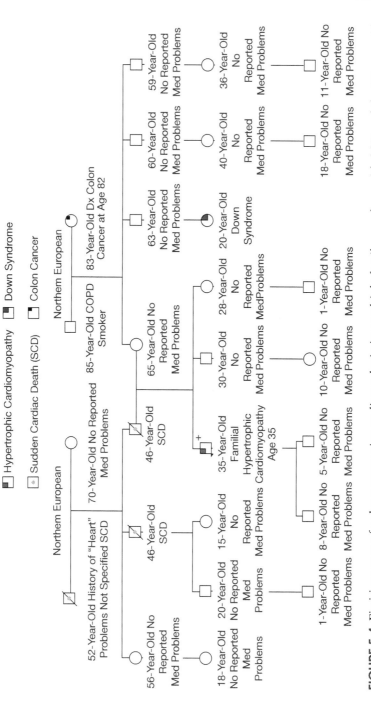

FIGURE 5.4 Fictitious case of a three-generation pedigree depicting multiple family members with SCD and the 35-year-old proband with a recent diagnosis of familial hypertrophic cardiomyopathy, an AD inherited condition.

AD, autosomal dominant; COPD, chronic obstructive pulmonary disease; Med, medical.

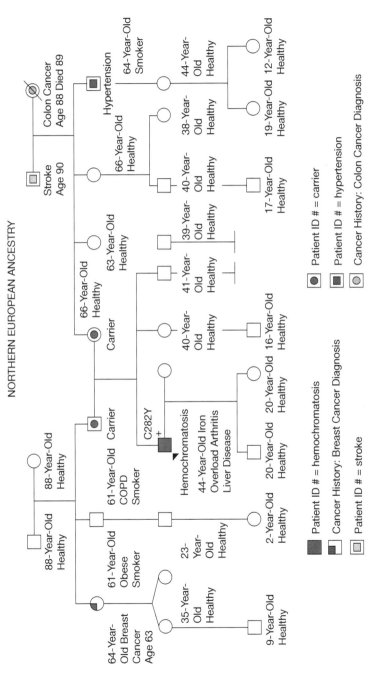

FIGURE 5.5 Pedigree (fictitious) of male proband (noted by arrowhead) diagnosed with hereditary hemochromatosis, an autosomal recessive disorder, with both parents being a carrier of the gene mutation but without disease.

COPD, chronic obstructive pulmonary disease.

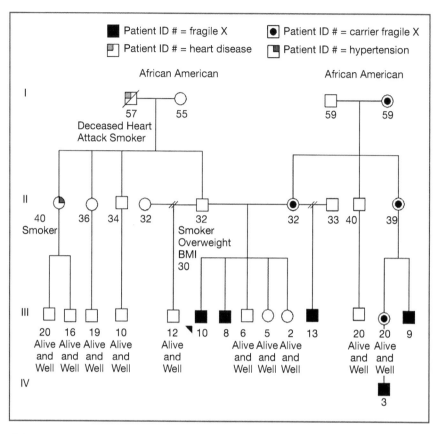

FIGURE 5.6 Fictitious pedigree with male proband and siblings, and other family members with fragile X syndrome, an inherited X-linked disorder.

BMI, body mass index.

Assessment and Interpretation of the Pedigree and Patterns of Inheritance

The three-generation pedigree provides an excellent means of observing relationships and patterns that may be suspect for an existing genetic disease or predisposition for disease occurrence. When the disorder is one of AD, *vertical transmission* can usually be observed in a pedigree with disease occurrence usually found in multiple generations. Figure 5.4 depicts a family history with multiple generations of individuals who died from sudden cardiac death (SCD) and the 35-year-old proband with recently diagnosed familial hypertrophic cardiomyopathy, an AD disorder. Note the vertical transmission of SCD in the paternal lineage.

In contrast to a pedigree depicting a family with an AD disorder like that noted in Figure 5.4, AR inherited disorders usually present on the pedigree as a *horizontal transmission*. The horizontal transmission appears to "skip" generations due to the fact that both parents must be at least carriers of the disorder. Figure 5.5 depicts a pedigree with hereditary hemochromatosis, with the male proband having the disease and both parents noted as carriers.

Note that in Figure 5.5 each of the specific disorders is represented in the legend and displayed differently by color or symbol. Individuals without disorders are presented here as "healthy." Also, the proband was

TABLE 5.2 Selected Online Resources for Family History and a Three-Generation Pedigree		
Online Resource	Description	Weblink
Centers for Disease Control and Prevention	Public health initiative to assist families with collecting and organizing their family history information	www.cdc.gov/genomics/famhistory/index.htm
National Institutes of Health, National Human Genome Research Institute	Offers a series of tools and guidelines to assess the family history	www.genome.gov/27527602
National Institutes of Health	An evaluation of the state of the science related to family history and its efficacy in practice	consensus.nih.gov/2009/Fhx%20images/family history_draftstmt.pdf
U.S. Surgeon General	Internet tool for consumers and health care professionals to build a simple pedigree	familyhistory.hhs.gov/FHH/html/index.html

tested for hemochromatosis, an AR disorder with the genetic findings included on the pedigree.

Besides AD and AR disorders, an X-linked pattern of inheritance can also be observed via a pedigree. Figure 5.6 depicts a three-generation pedigree of an affected male diagnosed with fragile X syndrome.

Once the information is collected and the pedigree is documented with the date of assessment, personal and family history should be addressed again during each patient visit to update the history regarding any pertinent changes. Be sure the initial date of the pedigree was recorded and the dates of any additional information are added to the original document. Failure to collect complete family history information from a patient compromises the clinician's ability to conduct an adequate genomic risk assessment, recognize patterns of disease inheritance, and provide appropriate counseling and strategies to manage care. Resources for the three-generation pedigree are presented in Table 5.2.

Info Box

A minimum of a three-generation pedigree provides an excellent tool to display the family history, enabling a visualization of patterns of inheritance if present that may aid in the recognition of genetic disorders. The pedigree should contain:

- Maternal and paternal lineages with ancestry of origin for each side of the family
- Designated proband or consultand emphasized (arrow)
- Appropriate nomenclature and standardized pedigree symbols
- Inclusion of all family members for three generations if known with age; current/past health status with pertinent medical and surgical history, and screenings/testing if applicable; and record of significant behaviors (e.g., smoking, alcohol use); include age of onset for medical and surgical history, and status—alive or deceased—including age and cause if known
- Legend for disease/disorders
- Date

Summary

Obtaining an in-depth family history, which includes a minimum of a three-generation pedigree, is an important step in the risk-assessment process. Conducting a family history, with that of other pertinent personal history data described in Chapter 4, enables health care providers, including APRNs, to obtain useful information in the recognition of potential red flags that may be suggestive of a genetic- or familial-related disorder. Chapter 6 continues the process of risk assessment by further describing interpretation of data to identify red flags that may warrant risk communication and management in the hopes of disease prevention, early diagnosis, and reduction of potential adverse outcomes due to disease occurrence.

References

Bennett, R. L. (1999). Getting to the roots: Recording the family tree. In *The Practical Guide to the Genetic Family History*. New York, NY: Wiley.

Bennett, R. L. (2010). *The practical guide to the genetic family history* (2nd ed.). Hoboken, NJ: John Wiley & Sons.

Bennett, R. L., French, K., Resta, R. G., & Doyle, D. L. (2008). Standardization human pedigree nomenclature: Update and assessment of the recommendations of the National Society of Genetic Counselors. *Journal of Genetics Counseling*, 17, 432–433.

National Coalition for Health Professional Education in Genetics. (2011). Core principles in family history. Retrieved from https://www.nchpeg.org/documents/NCHPEG%20FHx _CorePrinciples_31Aug11.pdf

National Heart, Lung, and Blood Institute. (2016, August 2). Who is at risk for sickle cell disease? Retrieved from https://www.nhlbi.nih.gov/health/health-topics/topics/sca/atrisk

Reid, G., & Emory, J. (2006). Chronic disease prevention in general practice—Applying the family history. *Australian Family Physician*, 35(11), 879–885.

Wilson, B., Carrol, J., Allanson, J., Little, J., Etchegary, H., Avard, D., . . . Chakraborty, P. (2012). Family history tools in primary care: Does one size fit all? *Public Health Genomics*, 15(3–4), 181–188. doi:10.1159/000336431

6

Step 2: Identification of Risk— Assessment of Red Flags

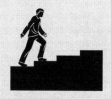 After completing the data collection process and reviewing the personal and family history, including pertinent tests and findings from the physical examination, all data should be synthesized and reviewed for *red flags* that are suspect for disease risk. The review may indicate frequent family members with chronic disease, which indicates a familial propensity or disease risk for the individual; alternatively, the reviewed data may be suspect for an inherited disease or genetic predisposition. The significance of risk assessment is *risk identification* so that appropriate measures can be implemented to reduce risk, establish the need for genetic testing if applicable, enable diagnosis, or institute prophylactic or treatment regimens to improve outcomes.

Objectives

1. Discuss red flags in the family history that may be suspect for a genetic predisposition to disease

2. Describe limitations in the family history regarding some genetic disorders

All data—personal and family history, physical examination as well as ancillary/radiology tests, and laboratory data, if applicable, obtained from the genomic risk assessment—should be carefully scrutinized to determine if there are elements for disease risk. Personal history issues that may be suspect for genetic disease include developmental delays, mental retardation, congenital anomalies, infertility, specific medical condition(s) or significant physical characteristics, and dysmorphology associated with inherited syndromes. Medical conditions associated with early-onset (e.g., colon cancer at age 35), atypical diseases based on gender or disease occurring in the less-often-affected gender (e.g., male breast cancer), rare cancers, and reproductive abnormalities such as recurrent pregnancy loss or infertility may raise suspicion for a genetic condition. Abnormal laboratory findings such as serum iron overload with elevated ferritin and transferrin saturation level or extreme lipid levels might suggest inherited hemochromatosis (autosomal recessive [AR] disorder) or familial hypercholesterolemia (autosomal dominant [AD] disorder), respectively. Physical examination findings, as previously stated, are also an important part of the genomic risk assessment as certain physical characteristics may be strongly suggestive of an inherited disorder. For example, sebaceous adenomas, epitheliomas, and carcinomas (Figure 6.1), as well as keratocanthomas, are all skin conditions that, if present and confirmed via clinical examination, may be suspect for an inherited colon cancer syndrome known as Muir–Torre syndrome, a form of Lynch syndrome (John & Schwartz, 2016; Mintsoulis & Beecker, 2016). Congenital hypertrophy of the retinal epithelium, a pigmented fundal lesion observed via ophthalmoscopic exam (Figure 6.2), may be observed in some individuals with familial adenomatous polyposis (FAP), an inherited colon cancer (Chen et al., 2006), and multiple café au lait spots on the skin or ophthalmic findings of Lisch nodules could be clinical signs of neurofibromatosis type 1 (*NF1*), an AD disorder (see Figures 6.1 to 6.3).

Family history is considered by some as the first genetic test. When complete and accurate, it can provide essential information that may denote patterns of inheritance indicating AD, AR, X-linked, or mitochondrial conditions. For example, a family history with unusual presentations like that of early age onset of sudden cardiac death may be suspect for an inherited cardiac disorder like familial dilated cardiomyopathy (80%–90% AD; rare AR and X-linked; U.S. National Library of Medicine [U.S. NLM], 2016), familial hypertrophic cardiomyopathy (AD), long

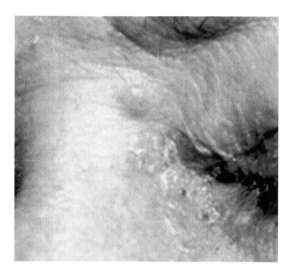

FIGURE 6.1 Sebaceous carcinoma of eyelid found during routine screening of a patient with Muir–Torre syndrome.

Source: Lynch and Anderson (2010).

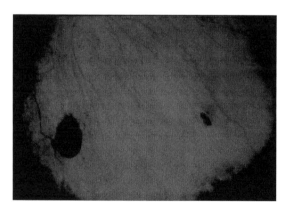

FIGURE 6.2 Congenital hypertrophy of the retinal pigment epithelium (CHRPE) that may be found in some patients with familial adenomatous polyposis (FAP), an inherited colon cancer disorder; it is not diagnostic of FAP.

Source: Half, Bercovich, and Rozen (2009).

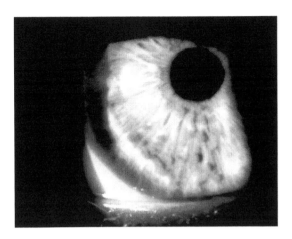

FIGURE 6.3 Multiple small, oval, yellow-brown papules (Lisch nodules) in the right iris.

Source: Adams, Stewart, Borges, and Darling (2012).

QT syndrome, or other hereditary cardiac conditions (Figure 6.4). It can also play an important role in determining above-average risk for disease based on *familial* risk, due to shared genetics and environmental factors. For instance, risk increases if more than one family member has the same illness, particularly regarding common chronic disorders such as diabetes, coronary heart disease, stroke, and some cancers (Acheson et al., 2010).

An early published mnemonic that can be used to identify red flags for genetic disorders is Family GENES, with the letter F and each letter in G-E-N-E-S representing elements that could be suspect for an inherited disease (Whelan et al., 2004). The F represents *family history*, denoting multiple family members with a specific disease or condition associated with a genetic syndrome that could indicate the need for further evaluation or genetic testing. A family history of multiple members in the family with colon cancer or colon and endometrial cancer, for example, might indicate a suspicion for Lynch syndrome. Table 6.1 shows some elements that denote red flags, including a brief description of the mnemonic Family GENES.

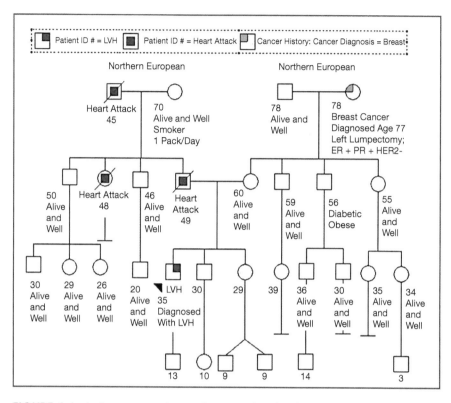

FIGURE 6.4 A three-generation pedigree with a family history suspect for early sudden cardiac death on the paternal lineage with the proband diagnosed at the time of hospitalization for left ventricular hypertrophy (LVH) attributed to a genetic cardiac disorder.

ER, estrogen receptor; HER2, human epidermal growth factor receptor 2; PR, progesterone receptor.

Limitations and Pitfalls of the History in Risk Identification

Although the personal and family history and physical examination play a critical role in determining genetic/genomic risk for disease, implementation of it does not guarantee identification of genetic red flags. Some examples of limitations from history data include inaccurate or unknown family history; adoption status; and AR pattern of inheritance that may

TABLE 6.1 Red Flags for Genetic/Genomic Conditions

Elements for Genetic Risk	Description or Examples
Family history-GENES[a] a. *Family history* b. *G* c. *E* d. *N* e. *E* f. *S*	a. Multiple *family members* with the same disorder or disorders associated with a syndrome b. Group of congenital anomalies c. Extreme or exceptional presentation d. Neurodevelopmental delays e. Extreme or exceptional pathology f. Surprising laboratory values (e.g., extremely high cholesterol levels)
Early age of onset of disease than is normally expected[b]	Colon cancer age 40; endometrial cancer age 40
Known genetic mutation in the family	Maternal aunt with a *BRCA* gene mutation
Certain physical exam findings (examples): a. *Café au lait spots* b. *Congenital hypertrophy of retinal pigment epithelium (CHRPE)*	Genetic disorder/syndrome a. Multiple spots may be suspect for NF1 b. Familial adenomatous polyposis—an inherited colon cancer syndrome
Ethnic predisposition to certain genetic conditions[b]	Sickle cell in African ancestry; *BRCA* germline mutations in Ashkenazi Jewish ancestry
Consanguinity[b]	Blood relationship with shared genes increases risk of autosomal recessive conditions
Recurrent pregnancy losses (two or more)[c]	Increase risk due to chromosomal anomalies
Disease in the absence of known risk factors[b]	Example of hyperlipidemia in an individual with normal weight, exercise

NF1, neurofibromatosis type 1.

Sources: [a]Whelan et al. (2004); [b]National Coalition for Health Professional Education in Genetics (NCHPEG; 2017); [c]Rull, Nagirnaja, and Laan (2012).

Genetic core competencies for advanced practice registered nurses (APRNs) include the ability to analyze a pedigree to identify potential inherited predisposition to disease and interpret the findings from the physical assessment, family history, laboratory findings, diagnostic tests, and/or radiology results that may indicate genetic/genomic disease, disease risk, or the need for a genetics/genomics referral (Greco, Tinley, & Seibert, 2012, p. 10).

not show disease occurrence in many generations due to the horizontal rather than vertical pattern of inheritance. In addition, genetics conditions impacted by *penetrance* and *de novo* mutations also influence the family history and may not result in identifiable red flags. *De novo* mutation is defined as a "new mutation" that is present for the first time in a family member as a consequence of a germline mutation in a germ cell or a mutation that arose during early embryogenesis (National Cancer Institute [NCI], n.d.). *Penetrance* refers to the likelihood that a clinical condition will occur based on the genotype (Cooper, Krawczak, Polychronakos, Tyler-Smith, & Kehrer-Sawatzki, 2013; NCI, n.d.). This means that the occurrence or signs and symptoms of disease is dependent on the genotype, with some genotypes having a high penetrance while others may have a reduced penetrance or probability of disease occurrence. For instance, gene mutations for FAP, an inherited colon cancer syndrome; multiple endocrine neoplasia; and retinoblastoma are complete (100%) penetrant disorders (Shawky, 2014), leading to disease certainty unless the individual dies of other causes. Although most inherited breast cancer syndromes are highly, but not 100%, penetrant, the risk for breast cancer is particularly high among those with a *BRCA* mutation, with an increased lifetime probability of breast cancer risk for women estimated at 50% to 87% (Antoniou et al., 2003; Ford et al., 1998). In addition, *variable expressivity* may lead to diagnosis failure, particularly with mild disease expressivity. Variable expressivity refers to the range of signs and symptoms that may occur from an inherited condition, which may vary from mild to severe and occur among individuals with the same genetic condition (NCI, n.d.). An example is the inherited condition of *NF1* that can manifest as café au lait spots only or severe disease with numerous neurofibromas and brain tumors

TABLE 6.2 Selected Online Resources for Red Flag Identification in Genomic Risk Assessment

Online Resource	Description	Weblink
National Coalition for Health Professional Education in Genetics With Agreement of the Jackson Laboratory—Clinical and Continuing Education	Online resource with numerous clinical topics related to using genetics in the clinic including risk assessment and identifying red flags and patterns that increase risk	www.jax.org/education-and-learning/clinical-and-continuing-education/family-history www.jax.org/education-and-learning/clinical-and-continuing-education/cancer-resources/cancer-risk-assessment
American Congress of Obstetricians and Gynecologists (ACOG)—Family History as a Risk Assessment Tool	ACOG Committee Opinion regarding family history as a risk assessment tool	www.acog.org/Resources-And- Publications/Committee-Opinions/Committee-on-Genetics/Family-History-as-a-Risk-Assessment-Tool
March of Dimes— Pregnancy and Health Profile	A screening and risk assessment tool	www.marchofdimes.org/materials/pregnancy-and-health-profile-a-clinical-assessment-and-screening-tool.pdf
Family Healthware™	A web-based research tool to assess a person's familial risk for six diseases (coronary heart disease, stroke, diabetes, and colorectal, breast, and ovarian cancers), providing users with a prevention plan for lifestyle changes and screening	www.cdc.gov/genomics/famhistory/famhist_healthware.htm www.familyhealthware.com/consumer

(NCI, n.d.). Further, *pleiotropy,* a single gene affecting multiple traits (Paaby & Rockman, 2013), may also result in different characteristics or clinical manifestations (phenotype) observed in the family history, making recognition and diagnosis of a genetic condition challenging if APRNs are not knowledgeable regarding this phenomenon. An example of pleiotropy is the multiple traits observed in mutations due to the cystic fibrosis trans-membrane conductance regulator (*CTFR*) gene that leads to AR cystic fibrosis disease (Cutting, 2015). Cystic fibrosis (CF) can have varied symptoms that can affect multiple organs (e.g., liver, sweat glands, pancreas, intestines), from life-threatening obstructive lung disease to atypical CF that is a milder form of the disease manifesting as chronic sinusitis and occurring later in adulthood (Schram, 2012) to other forms of CF such as male infertility due to bilateral absence of the vas deferens (Sokol, 2001).

Although there are some pitfalls and limitations in the history component of genomic risk assessment, the personal and family history, physical assessment, and integration of ancillary and laboratory data when applicable are the mainstay of determining disease risk. Table 6.2 is a list of resources that may be useful to identify red flags during the genomic risk assessment process.

Info Box

Although the personal and family history is the critical component of genomic risk assessment, *de novo* mutations, reduced penetrance, and variable expressivity could complicate identification of genetic disease.

Summary

The family history is an important part of the genomic risk assessment, as it provides essential information that may aid in identifying at-risk individuals for genetic disorders/syndromes or familial diseases. Clinicians, however, should be familiar with issues that make interpretation of the family history challenging to include faulty or unknown history, *de novo* mutations, reduced penetrance, variable expressivity, or genes that may cause multiple traits.

References

Acheson, L. S., Wang, C., Zyzanski, S. J., Lynn, A., Ruffin, M. T., IV, Gramling, R., . . . Nease, D. E., Jr. (2010). Family history and perceptions about risk and prevention for chronic diseases in primary care: A report from the Family Healthware™ Impact Trial. *Genetics in Medicine, 12,* 212–218.

Adams, E. G., Stewart, K. M., Borges, O. A., & Darling T. (2012). Multiple, unilateral Lisch nodules in the absence of other manifestations of neurofibromatosis type 1. *Case Reports in Ophthalmological Medicine.* Retrieved from https://openi.nlm.nih.gov/detailedresult.php ?img=PMC3350217_CRIM.OPHMED2011-854784.001&query=lisch+nodules&req= 4&npos=4

Antoniou, A., Pharoah, P. D., Narod, S., Risch, H. A., Eyfjord, J. E., Hopper, J. L., . . . Easton, D. F. (2003). Average risks of breast and ovarian cancer associated with *BRCA1* or *BRCA2* mutations detected in case series unselected for family history: A combined analysis of 22 studies. *American Journal of Human Genetics, 75*(5), 1117–1130.

Chen, C. S., Phillips, K. D., Grist, S., Bennet, G., Craig, J. E., Muecke, J. S., & Suthers, G. K. (2006). Congenital hypertrophy of the retinal pigment epithelium (CHRPE) in familial colorectal cancer. *Familial Cancer, 5*(4), 397–404.

Cooper, D. N., Krawczak, M., Polychronakos, C., Tyler-Smith, C., & Kehrer-Sawatzki, H. (2013). Where genotype is not predictive of phenotype: Towards an understanding of the molecular basis of reduced pentrance in human inherited disease. *Human Genetics, 132*(10), 1077–1130.

Cutting, G. R. (2015). Cystic fibrosis genetics: From molecular understanding to clinical application. *Nature Reviews, 16*(1), 45–56.

Ford, D., Easton, D. F., Stratton, M., Narod, S., Goldgar, D., Devilee, P., . . . Breast Cancer Linkage Consortium (1998). Genetic heterogeneity and penetrance analysis of the *BRCA1* and *BRCA2* genes in breast cancer families. The Breast Cancer Linkage Consortium. *American Journal of Human Genetics, 62*(3), 676–689.

Greco, K. E., Tinley, S., & Seibert, D. (2012). *Essential genetic and genomic competencies for nurses with graduate degrees.* Silver Spring, MD: American Nurses Association and International Society of Nurses in Genetics.

Half, E., Bercovich, D., & Rozen, P. (2009, October). Familial adenomatous polyposis. *Orphanet Journal of Rare Disease, 4*(22). Retrieved from https://ojrd.biomedcentral.com/ articles/10.1186/1750-1172-4-22

John, A. M., & Schwartz, R. A. (2016). Muir-Torre syndrome (MTS): An update and approach to diagnosis and management. *Journal of the American Academy of Dermatology, 74*(3), 558–566.

Lynch, M. C., & Anderson, B. E. (2010). Ileocecal adenocarcinoma and ureteral transitional cell carcinoma with multiple sebaceous tumors and keratoacanthomas in a case of Muir-Torre syndrome. *Dermatology Research and Practice.* Retrieved from https://openi.nlm.nih.gov/ detailedresult.php?img=PMC2931389_DRP2010-173160.001&query=muir+torre+syndrome& req=4&npos=2

Mintsoulis, D., & Beecker, J. (2016). Muir-Torre syndrome. *Canadian Medical Association Journal, 188*(5), E95. doi:10.1503/cmaj.150171

National Cancer Institute. (n.d.). NCI dictionary of cancer terms. Retrieved from https://www.cancer.gov/publications/dictionaries/cancer-terms?cdrid=446543

National Coalition for Health Professional Education in Genetics. (2017). Genetic red flags. Retrieved from https://www.jax.org/education-and-learning/clinical-and-continuing-education/cancer-resources/genetic-red-flags-checklist

Paaby, A. B., & Rockman, M. V. (2013). The many faces of pleiotropy. *Trends in Genetics, 29*(2), 66–73.

Rull, K., Nagirnaja, L., & Laan, M. (2012). Genetics of recurrent miscarriage: Challenges, current knowledge, future directions. *Frontiers in Genetics, 3*(34). doi:10.3389/fgene.2012.00034

Schram, C. A. (2012). Atypical cystic fibrosis. *Canadian Family Physician, 58*(12), 1341–1345.

Shawky, R. M. (2014). Reduced penetrance in human inherited disease. *Egyptian Journal of Medical Human Genetics, 15*(2), 103–111.

Sokol, R. (2001). Infertility in men with cystic fibrosis. *Current Opinion in Pulmonary Medicine, 7*(6), 421–426.

U.S. National Library of Medicine. (2016, October 4). Familial dilated cardiomyopathy. *Genetics Home Reference* [Internet]. Retrieved from https://ghr.nlm.nih.gov/condition/familial-dilated-cardiomyopathy

Whelan, A. J., Ball, S., Best, L., Best, R. G., Echiverri, S. C. Ganschow, P., Hopkin, R. J., Mayefsky, J., . . . Stallworth, J. (2004). Genetic red flags: Clues to thinking genetically in primary care practice. *Primary Care Clinics in Office Practice, 31*, 497–508.

7

Step 3: Selecting Risk Probability

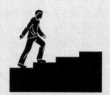 Once the data are assessed for elements of risk, or *red flags,* further evaluation should be conducted based on the identified risks to determine risk probability or empiric risk. Risk probability can be focused on the *genetic risk* based on the *probability or likelihood for an inherited disease or syndrome* or assessed for empiric risk regarding the chance of disease for noninherited diseases.

Does the collected and reviewed data suggest:

- Mendelian inheritance (autosomal dominant [AD], autosomal recessive [AR], X-linked)?
- *Familial* risk of chronic disease(s)?
- A family member with a known genetic mutation?
- *Population risk* based on uneventful data and no known risk factors?

Objectives

1. Differentiate between risk probability and empiric risk

2. Describe measures of determining risk probability as part of the genomic risk assessment

3. State evidence-based models that can be used as empiric risk models

Risk probability focuses on genetic risk or the probability or likelihood of an individual carrying a *genetic mutation* that further predisposes the individual for disease development (Baptista, 2005). *Empiric* risk is the chance of disease occurrence based on personal history, family history, or other important data. In the genomic risk assessment, evaluation of *risk* for the probability of having a genetic mutation that may predispose an individual to develop disease is as important as determination of disease risk based on noninherited disorders. Collected medical data, particularly the family history, play a key role in determining both genetic risk probability and empiric disease risk. Assessment of the family history for patterns suggestive of Mendelian inheritance may indicate the need to counsel the patient on genetic testing. A family history with a known genetic mutation may indicate a "high probability" of additional family members with the mutation based on the genetic disorder. The genetic disorder coupled with the individual's position in the family could also warrant the need for genetic counseling and the possibility of genetic testing for the patient. Figure 7.1 presents a fictitious case with a *high probability of a Mendelian genetic disease* suspect for an AD inherited breast cancer syndrome like hereditary breast and ovarian cancer (HBOC) based on the family history. Of significance is a family history of multiple female members with breast cancer in first-, second-, and third-degree relatives (proband, sibling, mother, aunts, grandmother), a male with breast cancer (cousin), a member with ovarian and breast cancers (grandmother), and early age onset of disease (age 40, breast; age 40, ovarian) on the maternal lineage. In another example (Figure 7.2), there is a single case of breast cancer without a well-defined pattern of inheritance; however, the limited family structure of few females and possibility of paternal inheritance, coupled with early age of onset of breast cancer (age 40) with triple negative disease, strongly suggests a high probability of a genetic inherited breast cancer syndrome based on personal history and the presence of red flags. In the previous hemochromatosis case (Figure 5.5), the male and female siblings may warrant counseling and genetic testing for the known mutation given that each sibling has a 25% risk of developing the disease as a result of the parent's carrier status as well as a 50% risk of himself or herself being a carrier of the disorder.

Although the history, especially that of the family, is the mainstay regarding genetic risk probability, there are prediction models to calculate genetic risk when a family history is suspect for specific inherited condition(s). *BOADICEA, BRCAPRO,* and *CancerGene* are examples of risk prediction models for the purpose of computing *BRCA1* and

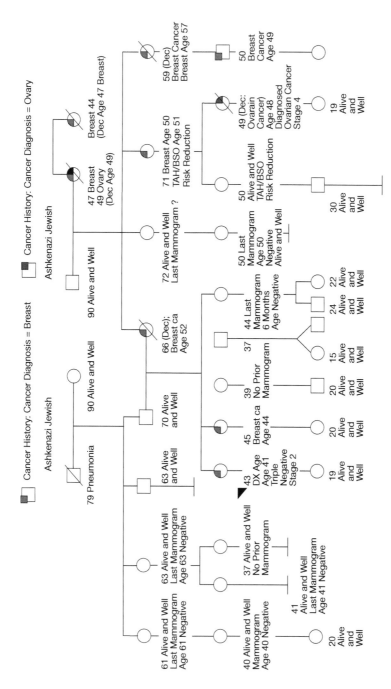

FIGURE 7.1 Fictitious pedigree with multiple family members having breast and/or ovarian cancer on the maternal lineage suspect for an inherited breast cancer syndrome. Note the vertical transmission.

ca, circa; Dec, deceased; DX, diagnosis; TAH/BSO, total abdominal hysterectomy and bilateral salpingo-oophorectomy.

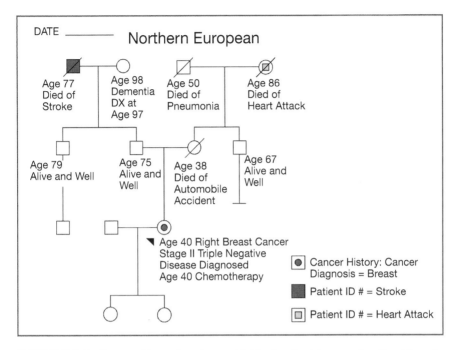

FIGURE 7.2 Pedigree with proband, age 40 (depicted with arrowhead) with early age onset of triple negative breast cancer (red flag) with limited family structure (e.g., few females on both maternal and paternal lineages and early age onset of death in mother limiting the ability to fully demonstrate observable pattern of inheritance).

DX, diagnosed.

BRCA2 mutation carrier probabilities for HBOC syndrome (Lee et al., 2014; Mazzola, Blackford, Parmigiani, & Biswas, 2015; UT Southwestern Medical Center, 2004). These models are used, if needed, with other data, especially that of family history for genetic risk prediction as noted. These models should be left to trained health care providers when applied to a clinical setting to ensure appropriate use and interpretation.

Chronic complex disorders are impacted by genetic, environmental, and behavioral factors. Personal, behavioral, familial, and environmental factors are all important when determining empiric risk estimates for many noninherited disorders. For example, having a first-degree relative with breast cancer nearly doubles a women's risk of developing the disease and having two first-degree relatives increases the risk almost threefold (American Cancer Society [ACS], 2016). This example denotes an *increased risk for breast cancer* even though the patient may have been assessed and found to have no mutation (*uninformative results*) through genetic testing (for more information on breast cancer, see Chapter 11). Similarly, the presence of a positive family history of cardiovascular disease (CVD) in the absence of genetic causation results in nearly a 40% risk increase of the disease in the siblings of an affected parent and 60% to 75% risk increase when the history is due to premature CVD (father younger than 55 years and mother younger than 65 years; Kolber & Scrimshaw, 2014). Modifiable (e.g., diet, tobacco use) and nonmodifiable (e.g., age, race/ethnicity, gender) factors can further increase an individual's empiric risk for disease occurrence for many conditions including both breast cancer and CVD. Evidence-based empiric risk models are available for many chronic disorders to estimate disease occurrence. For example, the Gail model is an empiric risk assessment tool that can be used to estimate a woman's (35 years of age and older) risk for breast cancer in the absence of a prior history of breast cancer, known gene mutation that elevates the risk for breast cancer, or prior history of mantle radiation for treatment of Hodgkin's lymphoma (National Cancer Institute [NCI], 2011). The 2013 cardiovascular risk calculator estimates individual's 10-year and lifetime risks for atherosclerotic CVD using age, gender, race, total cholesterol, high-density lipid (HDL) cholesterol, systolic blood pressure, blood pressure lowering medication use, diabetes status, and smoking status (American Heart Association & American College of Cardiology, 2016). It is important to remember, however, that when assessing an individual's risk based on *family history*, whether red flags exist that might indicate an inherited predisposition (genetic mutation) significantly increasing the risk of disease as well as other potential disorders depending on the genetic mutation. Individuals *suspect* (probability) for an inherited predisposition to disease should receive genetic counseling with consideration for genetic testing based on shared decision making and informed consent. Disease management if indicated is determined upon the presence or absence of the mutation (see Chapter 8).

For individuals with previously mentioned population risk based on empiric risk estimates, appropriate communication and management of risk should be provided based on the disorder. Risk for disease should be focused toward risk modification using medical and/or behavioral interventions that decrease risk (Baptista, 2005). Selected examples of online resources on risk assessment are presented in Table 7.1.

Info Box

Family history, preferably with a third-generation pedigree, is an important tool in assessing genetic risk probability for Mendelian disorders as well as empiric risk for disease development.

TABLE 7.1 Selected Online Resources for Risk Assessment

Online Resource	Description	Weblink
Empiric Risk Assessment Models		
Gail model	*Breast* Detailed description of the tool available. Not for women suspected of inherited disorder	www.cancer.gov/bcrisktool www.cancer.gov/bcrisktool/about-tool.aspx#gail
Claus	Use in women with a family history of breast cancer	young-ridge-2035.herokuapp.com
Framingham	*Heart* Gender-specific model that gives risk score for cardiac event	www.framinghamheart study.org/risk-functions/index.php www.framinghamheart study.org/risk-functions/cardiovascular-disease/index.php
2013 Cardiovascular Risk Calculator	Systematic cardiac risk charts based on European information	www.escardio.org/Education/Practice-Tools/CVD-prevention-toolbox/SCORE-Risk-Charts

(continued)

TABLE 7.1 Selected Online Resources for Risk Assessment *(continued)*		
Online Resource	Description	Weblink
Colorectal Cancer Risk Assessment	*Colon* Cannot estimate risk in high-risk categories (e.g., hereditary syndromes, ulcerative colitis, and Crohn's disease)	www.cancer.gov/ colorectalcancerrisk

Info Box

Personal history, physical examination, and additional personal data (laboratory, radiographs) with that of the family history can serve as important elements in determining risk probability "suspect" for an inherited disorder.

Summary

Careful review of personal and family history data is an important part of the risk-assessment process to determine if red flags exist that may be suggestive of an inherited disorder or syndrome. The use of empiric and/or risk-probability models, when available, may also aid in the risk-assessment process. This data can be useful in making decisions for further assessment, such as the need for genetic testing. A thorough and complete assessment of the data is important in determining risk probability, whether individuals are at population, moderate, (e.g., familial risk), or high risk (e.g., genetic mutation) for disease occurrence. Recognition of individual risk is essential in risk communication and risk management to prevent disease or reduce adverse outcomes.

References

American Cancer Society. (2016, June 1). What are the risk factors for breast cancer? Retrieved from https://www.cancer.org/cancer/breastcancer/detailedguide/breast-cancer-risk-factors

American Heart Association & American College of Cardiology. (2016). Prevention guidelines—2013 prevention guidelines tools CV risk calculator. Retrieved from http://professional.heart.org/professional/GuidelinesStatements/PreventionGuidelines/UCM_457698_Prevention-Guidelines.jsp

Baptista, P. V. (2005). Principles in genetic risk assessment. *Therapeutics and Clinical Risk Management*, *1*(1), 15–20.

Kolber, M. R., & Scrimshaw, C. (2014). Family history of cardiovascular disease. *Canadian Family Physician*, *60*(11), 1016.

Lee, A. J., Cunningham, A. P., Kuchenbaecker, K. B., Mavaddat, N., Easton, D. F., & Antoniou, A. C. (2014). BOADICEA breast cancer risk prediction model: Updates to cancer incidences, tumour pathology and web interface. *British Journal of Cancer*, *110*, 535–545.

Mazzola, E., Blackford, A., Parmigiani, G., & Biswas, S. (2015). Recent enhancements to the genetic risk prediction model BRCAPRO. *Cancer Informatics*, *14*(Suppl. 2), 147–157.

National Cancer Institute. (2011, May 16). Breast cancer risk assessment tool. Retrieved from https://www.cancer.gov/bcrisktool

UT Southwestern Medical Center. (2004). CancerGene. Retrieved from https://www4.utsouthwestern.edu/breasthealth/cagene

8

Step 4: Risk Communication and Risk Management

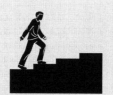 After all of the data are collected and evaluated, the next step in risk assessment is communicating the findings for the purpose of keeping the individual informed of his or her potential risk for an inherited disorder or chronic disease. Risk communication starts the process for appropriate risk management. Management is based on whether the individual is at population, moderate, or high risk (genetic disorder) for disease. If it is determined that the patient is suspect for a genetic disorder based upon his or her personal and/or family history, genetic counseling should begin, ensuring that ethical, legal, and social issues are considered. Genetic counseling often warrants referral to genetic professionals for further evaluation, pretest counseling if indicated, genetic testing, interpretation, and posttest follow-up for results and management of care.

Objectives

1. Discuss complexities of risk communication in patients suspect for an inherited disorder

2. Apply risk communication and risk management for a patient *above population risk* for a chronic disease

3. Describe ethical, legal, and social implications of individuals suspect for a genetic disorder

Once the genomic risk assessment process is completed and reviewed, communication of the results should be provided to the patient. What does the risk assessment process reveal regarding the patient's probability for a genetic disorder? Are there red flags warranting genetic counseling and consideration for genetic testing?

When the History Is Suspect for an Inherited Disorder

If the findings of the risk assessment process reveal that the individual is "suspect" for an inherited disorder, risk communication should begin. This risk communication process includes the need for genetic counseling and possibly genetic testing. For example, predictive and presymptomatic genetic testing can be used to detect if a genetic mutation exists that may not be present until later in life like that of most hereditary breast cancer syndromes (see Chapter 11). Carrier testing can identify individuals who may carry one copy of a gene mutation that can be important in preconception counseling and future pregnancy interest (see Chapter 9). Genetic testing can also be useful toward implementation of measures to reduce disease occurrence risk (e.g., chemoprevention or risk-reduction surgery for some individuals with breast cancer risk), determine management of care, and select therapeutic options such as occurs in surgical decision making (e.g., *BRCA* mutation positive patient with newly diagnosed breast cancer deciding on surgical options), as well as a means to monitor or treat disease. *Newborn screening,* for example, also involves a variety of genetic tests to identify genetic disorders in neonates that can be treated if detected early like phenylketonuria (PKU) and congenital hypothyroidism (see Chapter 10; Lister Hill National Center for Biomedical Communications, U.S. National Library of Medicine [NLM], 2017).

Patients who are suspect for a genomic disorder based on the assessment process should be informed of the assessment findings and the significance of the findings to a possible genetic disorder. The patient should be provided *genetic counseling* to discuss the potential of a genetic disorder, the availability of genetic testing, and potential consequences of positive results. According to the American Society of Human Genetics (n.d.), the goals of genetic counseling are to "assist the individual/family in understanding: (1) the diagnosis and implications of a condition; (2) the role of heredity; (3) recurrence risks and options; (4) possible courses of action; and (5) methods of on-going adjustment" (para. 3). The genetic counseling process involves interpreting and communicating complex information from the risk assessment process and how this information is associated with a potential genetic disorder and the need for genetic testing. The counseling process involves helping individuals make informed, independent decisions about their health care options, including genetic testing, while respecting the individual's beliefs, traditions, religion, family goals, and feelings (U.S. NLM, 2016). A genetic disorder, however, can affect various areas of one's life including financial, physical, social, medical, and overall quality of life. The need to consider ethical concerns is an important part of the counseling process pertaining to issues of confidentiality, insurance considerations, fear of discrimination, and employment (Bennett, 2010). The genetic counseling process should entail *pretest* and *posttest discussions, benefits* and *limitations of genetic testing, varied results* that may occur from genetic testing (e.g., mutation found; uninformative; variant of uncertain significance [VUS]), and *implication of results* regarding future management of care or risk management. The process is often complex, warranting genetic knowledge and skills from the advanced practice registered nurse (APRN) to avoid potential harm to the patient. Harm can be psychological, particularly when psychosocial issues of the disorder are not considered before testing, or physical as a result of incorrect testing or incorrect results interpretation. Therefore, the APRN must have knowledge and experience in genetics and genetic counseling to determine if testing is indicated; the type of test or tests to order; how to conduct genetic counseling including pre- and posttest counseling; a knowledge of the ethical, legal, and social implications of genetic testing; results interpretation; and in some cases who the appropriate family member is to test (e.g., informative member). These issues may even be more complex when children or minors are in need of testing, because the underage genetic testing of minors for adult-onset disease is not recommended in certain disorders like hereditary breast and ovarian cancer (HBOC; Charlisse, Caga-anan, Smith, Sharp, & Lantos, 2012) but may be required in cases like an inherited colon cancer syndrome such as familial adenomatous polyposis (FAP) where children may manifest with early age onset of the disease. Because of the myriad of knowledge and skills required for most genetic tests, we recommend referral to an individual expert in genetic testing (e.g., advanced genetics nurse [AGN], genetic counselor, medical geneticist) for further evaluation, counseling, and considerations for genetic testing.

Some health providers, including APRNs, may ask "why should one refer for genetic testing?" Let us look at some potential issues involved in genetic testing. First, genetic diagnosis can be complex as some disorders may involve numerous genes requiring correct decision making on what type of testing is indicated. For example, there are many genes that can cause hereditary colon cancer syndromes (see Chapter 11); therefore, genetic testing for some disorders can be challenging. Second, many genetic tests are not the same as other forms of laboratory testing where results may be clear and definitive. Important information to discuss with patients regarding genetic tests is what the results mean. In fact, certain genetic tests, while indicating no mutation found, may be uninformative in providing a reason for the personal or family history of disease unless a known mutation is noted to be in the family (e.g., a person with results indicating "no mutation" where a known mutation in the family is considered "negative"). Results may also reveal a VUS indicating that the variation in the genetic sequence and its association with disease is currently unknown and the finding cannot be classified as either pathogenic or benign. Individuals with a VUS on genetic test results often warrant future follow-up until the classification of the VUS is found to be pathogenic or benign. These findings may be misinterpreted by health care providers or others, resulting in inappropriate medical interventions or undue patient stress (Robson, Bradbury, Arun, Domcheck, & Ford, 2015). Uninformative or VUS results also warrant discussion of risk management (e.g., breast cancer, colon cancer, cardiovascular disease [CVD] risks) as testing was based upon the personal and/or family history that was *suspect* for an inherited predisposition to disease, meaning that despite an uninformative finding, the patient may still warrant significant management to prevent future risk of disease depending upon the personal/family history. Also, depending on the genetic disorder, mutation-positive test results may leave many unanswered questions as some genetic conditions may or may not lead to disease depending upon penetrance. Certain genetic disorders may have various means of disease presentation based upon their expressivity. Posttest counseling should include a detailed discussion of these issues as they relate to risk management and future management of care.

There are other issues to consider when ordering genetic tests. Because of the advances in technology regarding genetics, testing may involve numerous genes that predispose to a specific disease. For example, there are many germline mutations to consider when evaluating an individual for a colon cancer syndrome or a breast cancer syndrome. Genetic panel testing like that of *next-generation sequencing* (NGS) may be considered as a part of genetic testing for multiple syndromes that may cause a similar disease. These multigene panels can evaluate a large number of genes depending upon the genetic disorder evaluated. The use of the panels has a benefit in evaluating for a number of genes, enabling the potential for a quicker diagnosis and reducing or eliminating the need for the patient to have further testing; in addition, many multigene panels are cheaper when considering the cost of numerous single-gene tests. However, NGS or multigene testing has disadvantages. Because of the numerous genes tested, the possibility of one or more VUS findings may occur, leading to patient anxiety. In addition, *incidental unexpected* test findings may result, further causing anxiety and impacting future management of care that was not anticipated. Therefore, pretest and posttest counseling should be an integral part when considering genetic testing to discuss these issues and include an informed consent before testing (Robson et al., 2015).

The supportive, emotional element of risk communication is as important as the educational elements of risk communication (Edwards et al., 2008). The emotional element of genetic testing should be considered before ordering testing. People may feel angry, guilty, and/or depressed about the test results. Depending on the patient and genetic test, consideration for additional emotional counseling may be needed. In addition, fears of genetic discrimination or employment issues may also be concerning to patients. In 2008, the Genetic Information Nondiscrimination Act (GINA) was signed into law preventing discrimination against people based on their genetic information (National Human Genome Research Institute [NHGRI], 2012). This legislation bars health insurance companies and employers from discriminating against individuals on the basis of their genetic information. However, there are limitations to this law as individuals may be refused life insurance and long-term care insurance (NHGRI, 2012).

Family dynamics is another issue regarding genetic testing as positive findings often have implications for other members. Because of privacy issues, disclosure of results to other family members is the responsibility of the affected patient, warranting the health care provider to ensure the patient's understanding of the genetic results and implications to other family members. Some family members may have information they are reluctant to share that leads to dilemmas and ethical issues; thus, it is

TABLE 8.1 Examples of Genetic Counseling Resources and Referral Agencies

Resource	Description	Weblink
National Society of Genetic Counselors	Directory developed to assist health care providers in locating genetic counseling services	www.nsgc.org/page/find-a-gc-search
The American Society of Human Genetics (ASHG)	Mission is to advance human genetics in science, health, and society through excellence in research, education, and advocacy	www.ashg.org/education
American Board of Genetic Counseling	Includes consumer information on genetic counseling	www.abgc.net/Resources_Links/Consumer_Information.asp
GeneTests™ International Genetics Clinic Directory	Assists users in locating general and specialized clinical genetics services worldwide	www.genetests.org/clinics

important that the patient has a clear understanding of the genetic test results and implications to other family members if applicable regarding the patient's responsibility of results' sharing. Table 8.1 provides a list of genetic counseling resources for clinical practice when an inherited genetic condition and additional resources are needed.

When the History Indicates Above Population Risk (Nonhereditary)

Individuals frequently have a risk for a disorder based on personal life-style or behaviors, family history, or other environmental factors. Determination of risk is based upon data from the personal and/or family history. Risk communication and appropriate management of care should be initiated based upon the potential disease risk. For example, a

50-year-old White female of Northern European ancestry was recently diagnosed with *atypical hyperplasia* on breast biopsy; without a family history of breast cancer or other risks, she is at higher than population risk for developing future breast cancer. Using the Breast Cancer Risk Assessment Tool—Gail Model (National Cancer Institute [NCI], 2011), additional data regarding age of menarche (13), age of first live birth (25 years), family history of breast cancer in first-degree relatives (none), biopsy history (yes—one), and race/ethnicity (White) revealed a 5-year breast cancer risk of 2.5%, higher than that of an average woman of similar age (1.3%). The 2.5% risk is an estimated risk for her developing breast cancer in the next 5 years; her lifetime risk to age 90 was calculated at 21.3% higher than the 11.2% average risk for a woman of the same age (NCI, 2011). Based on her 5-year risk, the APRN now can discuss risk management that includes risk-reduction strategies such as chemoprevention (e.g., tamoxifen, raloxifene, anastrozole, exemestane), surveillance measures for early detection (e.g., mammography), weight management, and lifestyle modifications (e.g., physical activity, decrease alcohol consumption; Pruthi, Heisey, & Bevers, 2015).

Chronic diseases like CVD, diabetes, osteoporosis, and many cancers (e.g., colon) warrant assessment of risk so that preventative interventions can be implemented to reduce disease risks in the patient. Using the RISK acronym as a guide, the genomic risk assessment process can be used to assess an individual's risk for osteoporosis. The personal and family history is essential toward identifying elements of risk for osteoporosis. Risk factors for the disorder include a variety of modifiable and nonmodifiable factors. Specific risk factors for osteoporosis include female gender; advancing age; personal history of fracture after age 40; family history of osteoporosis; European or Asian ancestry; low body mass index or small, thin frame; diet and nutrition, particularly calcium and vitamin D deficiency; current cigarette smoking; certain medications; early menopause before age 45 years and estrogen deficiency; and certain medical conditions (National Osteoporosis Foundation, 2016; Rossini et al., 2016). Risk calculators for osteoporosis can also be used to further estimate empiric risk for the disorder and additional tools can be added to assess long-term fracture risk (e.g., FRAX; Briot et al., 2013; Rossini et al., 2016). Based on risk probability, risk management strategies can be discussed with the patient to reduce osteoporosis, fracture, and fall risks. Strategies could include primary prevention using medication (e.g., calcium), behavioral (e.g., physical activity), and lifestyle modifications to reduce falls as well as the incorporation of secondary measures via surveillance for early diagnosis (e.g., dual-energy x-ray absorptiometry [DEXA]).

When the History Indicates Average/Population Risk

Individuals are at risk for many diseases regardless of personal or family history. For example, the lifetime breast cancer risk for women is 12% even though the genomic risk assessment data are uneventful and without red flags. Even though the history data are normal, preventive measures to reduce chronic disease risks should be a part of normal clinical practice. Primary preventive measures such as age-appropriate immunizations and healthy lifestyles (e.g., physical activity; healthy eating; smoking avoidance; seat belt use) should be discussed during each patient visit. Appropriate secondary interventions like screening for early detection and diagnosis (e.g., Pap smear; mammography) should be ordered based on professional guidelines.

Info Box

Risk communication keeps patients informed about their likelihood or risk for disease occurrence based on personal and family history collected through the genomic risk assessment process. Risk communication is the initial step toward risk management where interventions can be discussed and implemented to improve health outcomes and reduce disease risk based upon the assessment data.

Summary

Patients need good information to make appropriate choices. Risk communication is a dialogue and information sharing process about the care options, including the harms and benefits of any intervention, which is particularly important when genetic testing is considered. Communication of risk is the first step toward providing risk management. The risk communication process should lead to greater mutual decision making and informed choices (Edwards et al., 2008; Fischoff, Brewer, & Downs, 2011). It should take account of individuals, age, attitudes, beliefs, culture, and religion. The use of risk communication and risk management can be an important measure in providing primary and secondary measures that incorporate chemoprevention, surveillance, risk-reducing surgery if applicable, and other strategies to reduce disease risk and improve health outcomes. Table 8.2 provides several resources to assist with the delivery of culturally sensitive genetic care; Table 8.3 provides some basic techniques that can be used for risk communication; and Table 8.4 provides additional genomic resources for use in risk communication and risk management.

TABLE 8.2 Genomic Resources for Cultural Communication

Online Resource	Description	Weblink
National Center for Cultural Competence (NCCC)	Online resource with consequences of care from both the patient and provider perspective	nccc.georgetown.edu/documents/FrontDesk Article.pdf
Genetic Counseling Cultural Competence Toolkit	Tips and tools for genetic counselors to enhance clinical skills	www.geneticcounselingtool kit.com/clinical_tools.htm
National Society of Genetic Counselors	Provides information on certified genetic counselors based on specialty and geographic location	www.nsgc.org
The American Society of Human Genetics	Online genetics education for health professionals	www.ashg.org/education/Health_Professionals.shtml

TABLE 8.3 Risk Communication Techniques

- Give the key messages and important information at the start of the communication.
- Speak to the patient about his or her rights and responsibilities.
- Shape the message to the needs of the patient:
  a. Relevant to patient needs
  b. Sensitive to the patient situation, beliefs, and culture
  c. Understandable in format and language
- Use pictures and stories for illustration if appropriate.
- Check patient understanding.

Source: Fischoff et al. (2011).

TABLE 8.4 Examples of Online Genetic Resources for Referral and Clinical Reference for Risk Communication and Risk Management

Genetic Resource	Description	Weblink
Genetic Testing Clinical Reference for Clinicians	American College of Preventive Medicine provides information on genetic testing time tool and clinical reference for clinicians	www.acpm.org/?GeneticTestgClinRef
GeneTests	Medical genetics information resource with information on genetic disorders, gene tests, laboratories, clinics, and other resources	www.genetests.org

References

American Society of Human Genetics. (n.d.). Genetic testing. Retrieved from http://www.ashg.org/education/genetic_testing.shtml

Bennett, R. L. (2010). *The practical guide to the genetic family history* (2nd ed.). Hoboken, NJ: John Wiley & Sons.

Briot, K., Patemotte, S., Kolta, S., Eastell, R., Felsenberg, D., Reid, D. M., . . . Roux, C. (2013). FRAX®: Prediction of major osteoporotic fractures in women from the general population: The OPUS study. *PLOS ONE, 8*(2), e83436. doi:10.1371/journal.pone.0083436

Charlisse, E., Caga-Anan, F., Smith, L., Sharp, R., & Lantos, J. (2012, January). Testing children for adult-onset genetic diseases. *Pediatrics, 129*(1), 163–167.

Edwards, A., Gray, J., Clark, A., Dundon, J., Elwyn, G., Gaff, C., . . . Thornton, H. (2008). Interventions to improve communications in clinical genetics. *Patient Education and Counseling, 71*(1), 4–25.

Fischoff, B., Brewer, N., & Downs, J. (Eds.). (2011, August). *Communicating risks and benefits: An evidence-based user's guide.* Silver Spring, MD: Federal Drug Administration and U.S. Department of Health and Human Services. Retrieved from http://www.fda.gov/downloads/AboutFDA/ReportsManualsForms/Reports/UCM268069.pdf

Lister Hill National Center for Biomedical Communications, U.S. National Library of Medicine, National Institutes of Health, Department of Health & Human Services. (2017, June 20). Help me understand genetics: Genetic testing. Retrieved from https://ghr.nlm.nih.gov/primer/testing.pdf

National Cancer Institute. (2011, May 16). Breast cancer risk assessment tool. Retrieved from https://www.cancer.gov/bcrisktool

National Human Genome Research Institute. (2012, March 16). Genetic Information Nondiscrimination Act (GINA) of 2008. Retrieved from https://www.genome.gov/24519851/genetic-information-nondiscrimination-act-of-2008

National Osteoporosis Foundation. (2016). Are you at risk? Retrieved from https://www.nof.org/prevention/general-facts/bone-basics/are-you-at-risk

Pruthi, S., Heisey, R. E., & Bevers, T. B. (2015). Chemoprevention for breast cancer. *Annals of Surgical Oncology, 22*(10), 3230–3235.

Robson, M. E., Bradbury, A. R., Arun, B., Domchek, S. M., & Ford, J. M. (2015). American Society of Clinical Oncology policy statement update: Genetic and genomic testing for cancer susceptibility. *Journal of Clinical Oncology.* doi:10.1200/JCO.2015.63.0996

Rossini, M., Adami, S., Bertoldo, F., Diacinti, D., Gatti, D., Giannini, S., . . . Isaia, G. C. (2016). Guidelines for the diagnosis, prevention and management of osteoporosis. *Reumatismo, 68*(1), 1–39.

U.S. National Library of Medicine. (2016, October 4). What happens during a genetic consultation? *Genetics Home Reference* [Internet]. Retrieved from https://ghr.nlm.nih.gov/primer/consult/expectations

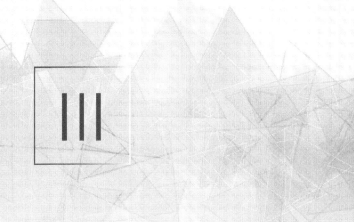

SPECIAL POPULATIONS

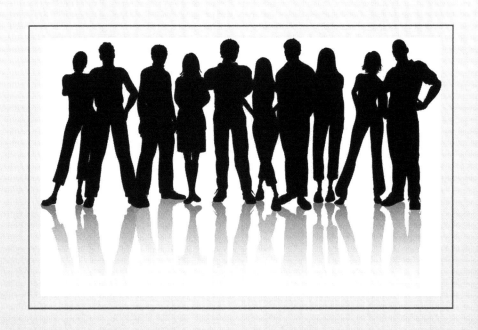

Chapters 9, 10, and 11 include the genomic risk assessment process as it relates to maternal/infant health; newborns, infants, and children; and cancer. The utilization of the acronym RISK is presented as it relates to evaluating individuals in each of these population categories during the risk assessment process.

Objectives for Part III

1. Differentiate the risk assessment process for each of the special populations

2. Identify genetic resources for each of the special populations

9

Risk Assessment in Preconception and Maternal Care

Jill Fonda Allen, Lisa M. Freese,
Quannetta T. Edwards, and Charles J. Macri

Genetics is the primary cause or plays an important role in many medical conditions and birth defects. Given that approximately 3% of newborns have a birth defect or genetic condition, many more develop significant conditions after birth, and more and more women with genetic conditions are having children, medical genetics is of prime importance in obstetric care. Evaluation of risk, identification of appropriate screening and testing options, and the ethical and psychological factors revolving around pregnancy may be encountered at any prenatal, preconception, or primary care visit for women of childbearing age and their families. It is essential that advanced practice registered nurses (APRNs) are knowledgeable about risk assessment and steps that follow when providing preconception and obstetrical (OB) care.

Objectives

1. Describe how RISK elements can be used when providing a genetic/genomic risk assessment for preconception care (PCC)

2. Discuss ancillary and laboratory measures in obstetrics that are used as part of the genetic risk assessment for screening and diagnosis of the fetus

99

The genomic risk assessment during preconception and prenatal care is more than evaluation of the risk for a single disorder; rather, it warrants a comprehensive assessment of medical, behavioral, environmental, and other factors that can impact maternal/infant outcomes. In this chapter, RISK elements are discussed as each applies to APRNs in conducting risk assessment when providing preconception or OB care. Before this discussion, Table 9.1 presents definitions of terms commonly used in obstetrics as it pertains to genetic testing.

Review of Data

Review of data as it relates to the personal history provides important information that can impact maternal/fetal outcomes prior to pregnancy. A comprehensive *personal history* should consist of (a) current age; (b) time period of pregnancy interest and age at time of expected delivery; (c) in-depth past and current medical and surgical history; (d) past and current medications including over-the-counter medications and contraceptives; (e) nutritional history; (f) lifestyle, behaviors, and environmental exposures;

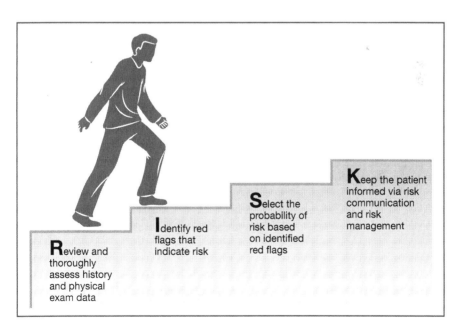

Preconception Care (PCC) and Risk Assessment

TABLE 9.1 Selected Terms Commonly Used in Obstetrics as They Relate to Genetic Assessment

Term	Description
Aneuploidy	Abnormality in the chromosomal number from the usual 46 (e.g., trisomy 21)[a]
Carrier screening	Screening conducted to identify individuals who have one copy of a gene mutation that, when present in two copies, causes a genetic disorder (e.g., autosomal recessive disorders)[b]
Noninvasive prenatal testing—after 10 weeks (10–22 weeks). Also known as cell-free DNA screening or aneuploidy	Cell-free DNA analyzed from the maternal blood for detection of pregnancies at increased risk for fetal aneuploidy and, if requested, sex chromosome composition[c, d]
Predictive testing	Testing used to detect gene mutations associated with disorders that usually occur later in life[b]
Prenatal diagnosis	Diagnostic testing done on fetal cells obtained from amniocentesis, chorionic villus sampling, or fetal blood sampling (rare) using varied techniques[b,e]

Types of prenatal testing
    Chromosome analysis
    DNA analysis
    Microarray analysis
	Testing that can be done on amniocytes, villi, or fetal blood to detect changes in the chromosomes or genes[b]

Preimplantation testing or screening (PGD and PGS)	Assessment of "embryos" (blastocysts) obtained via assisted reproductive measures (e.g., in vitro fertilization [IVF]) to detect genetic changes to allow transfer of an unaffected embryo to improve the success rate for IVF and/or to reduce the risk of miscarriage or of having an infant with a particular genetic or chromosomal disorder[b]

PGD, preimplantation genetic diagnosis; PGS, preimplantation genetic screening.

Sources: [a]Griffiths et al. (2000); [b]Lister Hill National Center for Biomedical Communications, U.S. National Library of Medicine, National Institutes of Health, Department of Health & Human Services (2017); [c]National Coalition for Health Professional Education in Genetics (2012); [d]American College of Obstetricians and Gynecologists (ACOG, 2015a); [e]ACOG (2014).

(g) psychosocial assessment; (h) immunization history; (i) prior gynecological and OB history including history of miscarriages, pregnancy outcomes during prenatal and postnatal period, as well as status of infant; and (j) reproductive plan. Undiagnosed, untreated, or poorly controlled medical conditions should be evaluated, including specific medications used and evaluation of teratogenic effects as should be employed as part of PCC and the risk assessment process (American College of Obstetricians and Gynecologists [ACOG], 2005; Nypayer, Arbour, & Niederegger, 2016). A comprehensive physical exam should be conducted and any abnormal findings that can impact maternal and fetal outcomes documented. Evaluation for infectious diseases (sexually transmitted infections) that can impact the pregnancy and neonate should also be conducted and pertinent counseling and management of care implemented. Carrier screening for genetic disorders (e.g., hemoglobinopathy, cystic fibrosis [CF] screen) is another important measure that should be offered based on the individual and partner's ancestry/ethnicity and family history. Sickle cell disease, for example, occurs more frequently in individuals of African descent with approximately one in 10 with the trait and one in 300 to 500 African American newborns with sickle cell disease (ACOG Committee on Genetics, 2017). Optimally, carrier screening should be part of PCC or the first OB visit. Carrier screening options should be based on professional guidelines from the ACOG and the American College of Medical Genetics and Genomics (ACMG). For example, individuals of Mediterranean, Asian, Middle Eastern, Hispanic, and West Indian descent are more likely to have mutations in beta thalassemia; alpha thalassemia is commonly found among individuals of Southeast Asian, African, West Indian, and Mediterranean ancestry. Currently, the ACOG Committee on Genetics (2017) recommends a complete blood count with red blood cell indices performed on all women to assess for anemia and hemoglobinopathies, with hemoglobin electrophoresis performed, in addition to complete blood count based on ethnicity described, if there is a suspicion for hemoglobinopathy (ACOG Committee on Genetics, 2017). In addition, CF carrier screening should be conducted for all women as part of PCC, or on women who are currently pregnant (ACOG Committee on Genetics, 2017). Carrier screening is discussed in more detail in the following.

Family history of the patient and her partner should be conducted and include preferably a three-generation pedigree (including siblings, niece/nephews, aunt/uncles, first cousins) to visualize potential relationships or patterns that may indicate genetic conditions. Assessment for the presence of mental retardation, birth defects, known or suspected hereditary conditions, or infant loss is central to determining what PCC genetic carrier screening should be implemented. Carrier screening is available for many autosomal recessive disorders (e.g., spinal muscular atrophy). A family history of mental retardation is an indication to offer fragile X carrier screening. Referral for genetic counseling should be made when further investigation is needed into the family history, when specialized carrier screening is warranted, or when one individual is identified as a carrier and carrier screening is needed on the partner.

Identification of Risk

Identification of risk should be based on information obtained from the comprehensive history. Table 9.2 provides a list of modifiable elements of risk or red flags based upon maternal history that warrant intervention.

Selecting the Probability of Risk

Selecting the probability of risk should be based upon identified risk factors (red flags) obtained from the history data and the evidence to support adverse outcomes to the mother and infant.

Keep the Patient Up to Date

Keep the patient up to date on data obtained from the history through risk communication and appropriate management of risk based upon identified red flags. Timely communication of results allows more time for follow-up (e.g., institution of folic acid supplements, or carrier testing of one's partner). Shared decision making that is culturally sensitive should be implemented with the goal of healthy maternal/infant outcomes. Although pregnancy outcomes cannot be guaranteed, providing evidence-based strategies should be communicated and implemented as part of PCC with the purpose of optimizing the chances for a healthy pregnancy and newborn.

TABLE 9.2 Elements of Modifiable Risk Based on Maternal History for Preconception Care

Potential Elements of Risk (Red Flags)	Interventions for Preconception Care
Unmanaged medical conditions (e.g., diabetes, hypertension)	Referral/consultation for management of care before pregnancy includes appropriate counseling of potential pregnancy risks
Current medication use with potential adverse fetal effects	Referral/consultation for possible medication substitution, change in dose, or reassurance regarding the relative safety of medical treatment
Nutritional deficiencies including overweight/obesity; underweight	Nutritional consultation a. Initiation of folic acid supplementation 1 month prior to pregnancy
Unhealthy behaviors or lifestyles (e.g., smoking, alcohol, drug use)	Management of behavioral risk before pregnancy attempt
Nonimmunized (e.g., rubella)	Immunization assessment and offer of vaccination counseling and immunize where applicable
Ancestry/heritage with specific carrier screening recommendations	Appropriate carrier screening or referral for genetic counseling
Family history of known or suspected genetic condition	Appropriate carrier screening or referral for genetic counseling

Application of Medical Genetics in Modern OB Care

Given the great number and wide variability of birth defects and genetic conditions, applying modern genetics to OB care is a challenge. It is necessary for OB care providers to be well versed with standard screening methods, integrate new screening options, be comfortable with prenatal diagnostic testing, and be familiar with specialized evaluation. It is also important for providers to be prepared to make appropriate referrals and know how to find genetic resources for their patients. This section focuses on practical application of these new and not-so-new developments.

Review History

An in-depth personal history is an important part of risk assessment and general OB/prenatal care. Current and maternal age at the time of delivery is important because advanced maternal age is a risk factor for Down syndrome, trisomies 13 and 18, as well as other maternal and fetal risks. Maternal age options are discussed in more detail under screening methods. Figure 9.1 presents a graphic display of the risk of trisomy disorders (aneuploidy) as a consequence of maternal age.

Besides age, the process of data review discussed previously for personal history may identify genetic risk factors. An in-depth OB history should also be obtained including history of abortions/miscarriages, fetal anomalies, or other conditions that impacted the infant at birth or later during childhood. Other factors important to the genetic history include environmental exposures related to employment (e.g., day-care provider's possible exposure to cytomegalovirus [CMV]), lifestyle (e.g., alcohol consumption), immunization status (e.g., rubella), medications (e.g., antiseizure), and travel history that may increase maternal/fetal risk (e.g., Zika virus). Questions should be carefully chosen to elicit a complete history. For example, "Have you or your partner traveled out of state or overseas in the past year? If yes, where did you travel? Did your travel(s) require premedication (e.g., antimalaria) or immunization(s)? Did you obtain the treatment or immunization prior to travel?" Although some of this inquiry may not directly relate to genetic disorders, the history may be important in order to differentiate inherited or chromosomal disorders from other environmental factors if a problem is found during or immediately after the pregnancy.

A family history should be taken to screen for genetic risk factors. Having the patient complete a family history questionnaire prior to the visit may help start this process. My Family Health Portrait, available via familyhistory.hhs.gov, is one resource that family members can use to obtain data relating to the family history. However, a personal interview will prompt a more complete history that might lead to discovery of a risk for inherited conditions. The family history should include general and

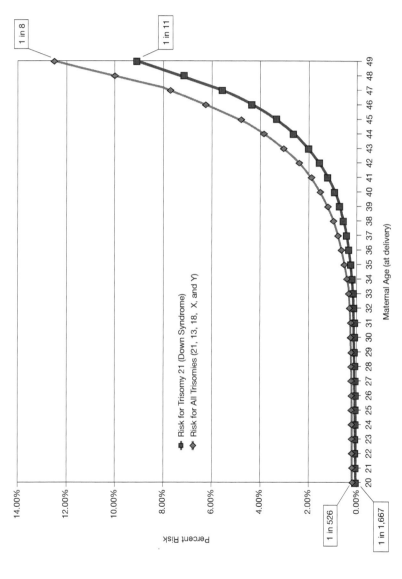

FIGURE 9.1 Risk for trisomy disorders based on advanced maternal age.

Sources: Egan (2004); Hook, Cross, and Schreinemachers (1983); Newberger (2000).

specific inquiry about the health of immediate family members (children, siblings, and parents) and at least general and preferably specific inquiry regarding second-degree relatives (aunts, uncles, and cousins). General inquiry has been shown to be ineffective in identifying all potential risks, as patients may not consider a relative to have "mental retardation" or "birth defects" that could be attributed to inherited disorders (particularly recessive or X-linked disorders). Asking questions from the patient's perspective, using nonmedical terminology such as "Were there any infants in the family history who did not survive or needed surgery at birth?" or "Were there any individuals who were not independent as adults?" might be more effective in obtaining a relevant history and elicit red flags that may be attributed to inherited or chromosomal disorders.

Identify Red Flags Through Screening Methods

The personal and family history is one way of identifying red flags that may suggest a risk for genetic disease, chromosomal disorders, or other potential risks to the fetus. However, there are a number of screening tests that may be done on a standard basis during pregnancy and other tests available for high-risk situations to evaluate the fetus's status or well-being. These can generally be divided into screening tests and diagnostic tests. It is important to discuss these tests in advance with patients and clarify with them the purpose, limitations, and optional nature of each of these tests. This pretest discussion should be geared to enable informed consent and prepare patients for potential results. Approaching evaluation for possible genetic risk factors from a chronological standpoint during pregnancy provides a logical and practical framework for the practitioner. Most of the following tests should be offered based on the ACOG and the ACMG guidelines. Initial discussion should take place prior to or very early in pregnancy, preferably by 8 weeks gestation, to allow the patient time to consider and then schedule testing.

Genetic carrier screening should be offered to all patients based on the patient's ancestry, heritage, or ethnicity as increased frequency of some genetic diseases is found to occur in higher rates among certain groups (Edwards, Seibert, Macri, Covington, & Tilghman, 2004; Nazareth, Lazarin, & Goldberg, 2015). It is important to assess ancestry/ethnicity for both the maternal and paternal lineages at the time of the preconception or initial obstetrics visit. As noted previously, ACOG/ACMG guidelines should be followed. For example, carrier frequency of Tay–Sachs disease, a severe progressive neurologic disease that causes death in early childhood, is one in 30 for Ashkenazi Jewish ancestry, compared to one in 300 in non-Jewish populations, with French Canadians and individuals of Cajun descent having higher frequency rates compared to general population (ACOG Committee on Genetics, 2017; Park et al., 2010). Tay–Sachs carrier screening using either DNA-based testing/mutation analysis or biochemistry (Hex A) should be offered to women who are or whose partner is of Ashkenazi Jewish or half Jewish ancestry, even if she or her partner is not. In addition, the ACOG Committee on Genetics (2017) recommends that carrier screening for Canavan disease, CF, and familial dysautonomia (using DNA) and other disorders should be discussed and offered to individuals of Ashkenazi Jewish descent. Carrier screening for alpha thalassemia should be offered to individuals of Asian heritage, especially those with anemia or conditions where the red blood cell size (MCV) or hemoglobin amount relative to the size of the cell (MCH) is low. CF is more common among non-Hispanic Whites compared with other racial/ethnic groups with a carrier frequency of one in 25; however, because of difficulty in assigning the disorder to one specific ethnic group, screening for CF is reasonable for all couples according to the ACOG Committee on Genetics (2017). It can be a challenge for the practitioner to stay current with genetic carrier screening practice guidelines, as the number and nature of carrier screening options changes with new advances (e.g., expanded carrier screening [ECS] panels).

Genetic carrier screening should be offered or a referral for genetic counseling to explore possible carrier screening should be made as indicated based on family history (e.g., if a family member is diagnosed with a specific condition or is known to be a carrier for a genetic condition). The presence of a family member with mental retardation or autistic spectrum disorders should prompt a discussion of fragile X carrier screening. Also, as per the ACOG and the ACMG, individuals with a family history of birth defects, mental retardation, or recurrent miscarriage should also be offered chromosome analysis to exclude carrier status for a chromosome rearrangement (translocation).

Availability of ECS panels (multiple genetic carrier screening tests) is another carrier screening option that patients may consider. These panels are generally not based on ethnicity or family history and may be offered to any interested individual with complete informed consent. However, ECS panels may also be offered based upon personal and/or family history (Wienke, Brown, Farmer, & Strange, 2014). For example, some of these panels include DNA-based carrier screening for recessive genetic disorders seen with more frequency in the Ashkenazi Jewish population (Canavan disease, CF, familial dysautonomia, and Tay-Sachs). Also, recommendations for more comprehensive screening have been made for individuals of Ashkenazi Jewish descent to include a host of other conditions, which include Bloom syndrome, familial hyperinsulinism, Fanconi anemia, Gaucher disease, and Niemann-Pick disease, as well as other diseases (ACOG Committee on Genetics, 2017). Health care providers caring for these high-risk individuals in this racial/ethnic group may want to refer for genetic counseling to ensure appropriate genetic screening is considered. ECS panels may also be appropriate for consanguineous couples (first cousins), by testing for a larger group of recessive conditions. However, the efficacy of ESC panels has yet to be determined. In one study, the carrier frequency of more than 100 genetic mutations for 16 recessive disorders was nearly 1:3.3 for one disorder and one in 24 for two disorders among Ashkenazi Jews (Scott et al., 2010). Outcome-based studies that focus on identification of carrier couples (not just carriers) are needed to establish the efficacy of these panels, not only from a cost perspective, but also from patient and provider perspectives. Some organizations provide targeted carrier screening programs at reduced cost or on college campuses (e.g., Jewish heritage or sickle cell carrier screening). The potential impact of identifying couples who are both carriers for these recessive genetic diseases is one more example of the importance of the genetic risk assessment in preconception and prenatal care.

During pregnancy, other factors may prompt a need for referral for genetic counseling, screening, or prenatal diagnosis. Maternal age is an indication for in-depth discussion and genetic counseling regarding associated risks and options for screening or prenatal diagnosis. This discussion may be valuable for families planning future pregnancies, as maternal age–related risks may prompt them to have children closer together after 35 years of age, or take birth control more seriously after they have completed their family. The complexity of maternal age screening and prenatal diagnostic testing options and personal nature of choices regarding these tests warrants formal genetic counseling. However, a summary of current options for standard screening available in any pregnancy including those with advanced maternal age follows. Prenatal screening tests "show only whether a woman is at low or high risk for having an infant with a particular disorder" (ACOG, 2015b, para. 2), but may be used to guide decisions regarding prenatal diagnosis. Examples of current tests are described in the following.

First-trimester screening is the earliest test currently offered to screen for Down syndrome (trisomy 21), trisomy 18, and trisomy 13. It is also effective in recognizing or suspecting certain major fetal anomalies (e.g., anencephaly) well in advance of the formal detailed ultrasound at 18 to 20 weeks. This means that a woman whose fetus has major anomalies is now often alerted to their presence at the end of the first trimester, allowing much earlier patient–provider shared decision making regarding possible pregnancy termination or expectant care for these lethal anomalies. A summary of first trimester and other prenatal screening measures are presented in Table 9.3.

Another more recent prenatal screening option is the use of cell-free DNA (cfDNA) screening for aneuploidy, also referred to as *noninvasive prenatal screening* (NIPS). cfDNA screening can detect women at increased risk for Down syndrome, trisomies 13 and 18, and, if desired, determine fetal sex (Thompson, 2015). This screening test involves the use of cfDNA from pregnant women taken via from the mother's blood at or after 10 weeks gestation and is not a routine test nor currently recommended as a first screening test in low-risk or multiple pregnancies (ACMG, 2016; ACOG, 2015b; Thompson, 2015). According to the ACMG (2016), the NIPS is the "most sensitive screening option for traditionally screened aneuploidies involving chromosomes 13, 18, and 21" (para. 4). The cfDNA is currently used to detect aneuploidy (trisomies 21, 18, and 13) and does not detect other chromosome abnormalities or fetal anomalies (e.g., spina bifida and other neural tube or abdominal wall defects), and conventional screening methods discussed previously remain the most appropriate choice for prenatal screening for these conditions in low-risk populations. However, cfDNA may be the most appropriate screen for women at increased risk for fetal aneuploidy, especially when used in conjunction with conventional screening methods (Allen, Stoll, & Bernhardt, 2016). As part of informed consent, patients should have precounseling prior to undergoing cfDNA or any screening test to ensure that they understand that a negative result does not ensure an unaffected pregnancy and any positive test warrants further evaluation to exclude a false positive (ACOG, 2015a; Allen et al., 2016). It is important that referral to a trained genetics professional be made to all patients with a positive

TABLE 9.3 Common Prenatal Screening Tests for Birth Defects

Prenatal Screening Test	Purpose
First-trimester screening[a,b,c] • Serum pregnancy-associated plasma protein-A (PAPP-A) and human chorionic gonadotropin (hCG) and ultrasound examination for nuchal translucency (NT)	• Down syndrome • Trisomies 13 and 18 • Very early anatomy for major anomalies and suspicion of cardiac defects, other possible defects
Second trimester: Maternal serum alpha-fetoprotein (MSAFP) • Serum AFP, only[b]	• Neural tube defects including spina bifida and anencephaly, as well as abdominal wall and other possible defects
Second trimester: AFP quad/tetra screen[b] • AFP, hCG, estriol, and inhibin A	• Neural tube defects including spina bifida and anencephaly • Down syndrome • Trisomy 18 • Similar to AFP screen between 15 and 20 weeks of pregnancy for patients who do not present early enough in pregnancy or miss the window for the first-trimester screening

Ultrasound
• *Markers*:
  NT
  (11–13 weeks, 6 days)[c]
  her markers for possible Down syndrome[f] (optimal 18–21 weeks)
  • Shortened femur or humerus; absent nasal bone; pyelectasis; intestinal hyperechogenicity; single umbilical artery
	• Fetal thickening of the neck area with fold measuring ≥ 2.5–3 mm at 11–14 weeks: marker for Down syndrome[d]

Sources: [a]Spaggiari et al. (2016); [b]American College of Obstetricians and Gynecologists (ACOG, 2014); [c]Guraya (2013); [d]Renna et al. (2013); [e]Souka, Von Kaisenberg, Hyett, Sonek, and Nicolaides (2005); [f]Kataguiri et al. (2014).

cfDNA/NIPS or first-trimester screening result so that further counseling and diagnostic testing can be offered (ACMG, 2016).

In addition to these screening methods, ultrasound assessment of fetal anatomy for anomalies and *markers* (Table 9.3) remains an invaluable tool for prenatal diagnosis of fetal anomalies and to screen for Down syndrome and other genetic conditions. Standard screening is done in conjunction with first-trimester screening between 11 and 13 weeks 6 days, and again for full anatomical evaluation at 18 to 21 weeks gestation. Suspicion of certain conditions based on ultrasound findings often prompts consideration of further testing such as chorionic villus sampling (CVS) or amniocentesis to enable chromosome, DNA, or microarray analysis to confirm a suspected diagnosis. The concept of dysmorphology, differences in physical form, used in pediatric genetics to evaluate infants and children with suspected genetic conditions can be readily applied to ultrasound. A central concept in dysmorphology is that a single birth defect is often an *isolated birth defect,* but an infant with multiple findings often has a generalized condition, such as a chromosome abnormality or genetic syndrome. With this same logic, the finding of a birth defect or "marker" on prenatal ultrasound should prompt further fetal evaluation and review of other risk factors that may provide evidence or clues to the presence of a more complex condition. When ultrasound evaluation or any of the previously mentioned standard prenatal screening tools identify a birth defect or marker, prompt referral for further evaluation (e.g., high-resolution ultrasound, fetal echo, or MRI), and possible prenatal diagnosis via CVS or amniocentesis, and consultation with a genetic counselor or other genetic or pediatric specialists should be made (Dey, Sharma, & Aggarwal, 2013).

Selective Tests Based on Red Flags: Invasive Procedures and Prenatal Diagnosis

Prenatal diagnosis using invasive procedures like amniocentesis or CVS should be offered based upon maternal age older than 35 at delivery, any of the screening test results that show an increased risk for a birth defect, or parents with risk factors that increase the risk of having an infant with certain birth defects. However, the ACOG (2015b) notes that "screening and *diagnostic tests can be offered to all women regardless of history*" (para. 4). Table 9.4 provides examples (not all exclusive) of reasons for offering invasive prenatal testing.

TABLE 9.4 Common Reasons for Offering Invasive Prenatal Testing

- Woman age 35 or older at expected time of birth
- Woman who carries an X-linked genetic abnormality such as Duchenne or Becker muscular dystrophy, fragile X syndrome, or hemophilia
- Fear of having a child with a chromosome or microarray abnormality
- Prior child with chromosome or microarray abnormality or metabolic abnormality (inborn error of metabolism)
- Prior child with developmental abnormality
- Prior child with structural abnormality associated with a malformation or genetic or chromosomal abnormality (e.g., spina bifida)
- Parents are both carriers for autosomal recessive genetic disorder (e.g., Tay–Sachs disease, sickle cell anemia)
- A parent who is a carrier of a chromosome rearrangement such as a translocation
- Ultrasound finding of structural abnormality
- Abnormal first-trimester screening
- Abnormal second-trimester screening
- Abnormal maternal serum alpha-fetoprotein (MSAFP)
- Risk of viral illness (Zika, CMV, Rubella, etc.)

CMV, cytomegalovirus.

Prenatal diagnostic testing via an amniocentesis, the most common procedure for prenatal diagnosis of inherited conditions, is typically performed between the 15th and 20th weeks of pregnancy but can be performed outside this time frame when indicated. It is performed to obtain amniotic fluid and the amniocytes (cells of fetal origin) contained in the fluid. CVS is performed primarily between 10 and 13 weeks of pregnancy to obtain chorionic villi (placental tissue). Cells obtained via amniocentesis or CVS may be used to identify *chromosomal abnormalities* as well as *genetic mutations.* The commonly used tests conducted for genetic disorders using fetal cells obtained from these prenatal tests include *karyotype* (microscopic chromosome analysis including number and structure), amniotic fluid alpha-fetoprotein (AFAFP) analysis, and fluorescence in situ hybridization (FISH). More recently, the use of chromosome microarray (CMA) analysis for detection of submicroscopic copy number variants (CNVs) has become available and should also be discussed with any patient undergoing invasive prenatal diagnostic testing. Microarray analysis, DNA analysis, and biochemical analysis (ACOG, 2015b) may also be indicated in specific situations. Amniotic fluid samples may be analyzed using certain biochemical or viral tests in specific situations (e.g., CMV or Zika virus). It may be overwhelming for patients whose pregnancies have been identified to be at increased risk to process all of these options and make informed decisions. Genetic counseling prior to prenatal testing is indicated to enable informed consent by the patient for testing, and should include discussion of the purpose, accuracy, and limitations of each test being offered or performed.

Specialized Testing

As research and clinical advances continue, the number and complexity of testing options continues to expand. FISH is a method used to rapidly detect common fetal aneuploidies found at the time of prenatal invasive testing using fluorescent-tagged probes for the most common fetal chromosome aneuploidies (trisomies 13, 18, 21, X, Y, and triploidy; Norwitz & Levy, 2013). Specialized FISH techniques may be used to detect certain other conditions (e.g., DiGeorge syndrome: microdeletion 22q).

Chromosomal microarray analysis (CMA) for prenatal diagnosis uses specialized DNA methods to identify chromosomal abnormalities that are too small to be identified via conventional chromosome analysis (karyotype), including submicroscopic deletions and duplication referred to as CNVs. Specifically, it measures gains and losses of DNA throughout the human genome, enabling identification of chromosomal aneuploidy and location and type of certain genetic changes (ACOG, 2013; Society for Maternal–Fetal Medicine [SMFM], Dugoff, Norton, & Kuller, 2016). CMA has limitations, as it cannot detect most single-gene changes. CMA may also identify small losses or gains of genetic material for which the clinical significance is uncertain or unknown. These findings are referred to as variants of unknown significance (VUS, see Chapter 2 for definition of VUS). Indications for the use of CMA in prenatal diagnosis include ultrasound finding(s) suggestive of fetal structural anomalies, intrauterine fetal demise or stillbirth, or prior child with a microarray abnormality. However, patients with a structurally normal fetus undergoing invasive prenatal diagnostic testing should be informed of the availability and limitations of CMA and offered either conventional karyotyping or CMA (ACOG, 2013; SMFM et al., 2016). Parents who request this testing without a specific diagnosis should speak with their doctor or a genetic counselor to discuss the potential benefits, limitations, and possible results in advance of testing.

Additional Alternatives

Some families at risk for genetic conditions may take alternative approaches. These include *preimplantation genetic screening* (PGS) or diagnosis (PGD) in conjunction with in vitro fertilization (IVF). Individuals may undergo *predictive testing* for adult onset conditions in advance of family planning. Couples may also choose to use a gamete donor or surrogate depending upon their personal/family history and risk for a genetic condition.

Keep Patient Informed: Risk Communication and Management via Genetic Counseling

Risk communication and management are important parts of preconception and prenatal screening and diagnostic testing. Genetic testing results may have significant implications for medical management and personal decision making as well as implications to other family members or future pregnancies. It is imperative that providers enable informed decision making and allow informed consent by providing comprehensive counseling prior to genetic carrier testing and prenatal screening or diagnosis. This may be done by a generalist. However, many of the procedures described previously (e.g., CVS, amniocentesis) warrant specialized care by a perinatologist. A genetic counselor might be needed for fully informed consent and decision making, as well as to coordinate specialized genetic testing. Knowledgeable providers should oversee the ordering of genetic tests. The skills and training of a board-certified advanced genetics nurse (AGN), as well as certified genetic counselors or geneticists, are often necessary to complete the genetic counseling process. For example, comprehensive patient pretest and posttest genetic counseling by a "qualified" provider should be involved in patients undergoing CMA with discussion and documentation in the medical records of potential for VUS, nonpaternity, consanguinity, and adult-onset diseases with informed consent completed (ACOG, 2013; SMFM, 2016).

Invasive prenatal diagnostic tests like CVS and amniocentesis are performed by physicians, typically a perinatologist or maternal–fetal medicine specialist, with expertise in this area. Counseling with informed consent on these procedures should also be conducted prior to the procedure to include discussion of potential risks and possibility of ambiguous results (e.g., maternal contamination and mosaicism with CVS). Pretest and posttest counseling should be conducted by individuals with expertise, and patients with abnormal or ambiguous findings should always be referred to the appropriate specialist or specialty team for management of care (e.g., neonatologist, perinatologist, fetal therapy, or management program). Given the complexity of issues and the time-consuming nature of this process, referral to a genetic counselor or AGN may be an appropriate step in the genetic testing process.

Genetic counseling is a process and includes: (a) interpretation of family and medical histories to assess risk of disease occurrence or reoccurrence; (b) education about inheritance, testing, management, prevention, resources, and research; and (c) counseling to promote informed choices and adaptation to the risk (National Society of Genetic Counselors [NSGC], n.d.-a). Prenatal genetic counseling refers to both preconception and prenatal care where applicable. Genetic counseling is often, but not always, provided by a certified genetic counselor. Table 9.5 provides a composite summary of reasons for prenatal genetic counseling

TABLE 9.5 Reasons for Referral for Individuals for Preconception or Prenatal Genetic Counseling

- Women or couples interested in screening or diagnostic testing for a current or future pregnancy (preconception)
- Maternal age 35 or older at time of delivery
- Multiple gestations
- Abnormal results for prenatal screening tests, ultrasound, or other testing
- Abnormal testing from diagnostic testing (e.g., CVS or amniocentesis)
- Individuals of racial/ethnic groups with high rates of inherited diseases (e.g., Jewish; French Canadian; Asian backgrounds)
- Women exposed to certain medication, drugs, radiation, or infection
- Women with history of multiple miscarriages or infertility
- Women or couples with known carrier of a genetic condition
- Known consanguinity
- Personal diagnosis, previous child, or family history of birth defect, genetic disorder, or mental retardation

CVS, chorionic villus sampling.
Source: NSGC (n.d.-b).

TABLE 9.6 Selected Online Resources for Prenatal Genetic Risk Assessment

Online Resource	Description	Weblink
GeneTests	Medical genetics with laboratory directory; clinic directory for diagnosis and genetic counseling service and links for disorders and genes	www.genetests.org
Genetic Disease Foundation	Nonprofit organization with mission to support research, education, and prevention of genetic diseases	ghr.nlm.nih.gov/condition
Genetics Home Reference	U.S. National Library of Medicine—health conditions including signs and symptoms, frequency, genetic cause, and inheritance patterns of diseases and syndromes	www.genome.gov/10001204/specific0genetic-disorders
Learning About Specific Genetic Disorders a. Tay–Sachs disease b. Down syndrome	National Human Genome Research Institute with list of selected genetic diseases a. Information about Tay–Sachs disease include testing and resources b. Information about Down syndrome including testing and resources	www.genome.gov/10001220/learning-about-taysachs-disease www.genome.gov/19517824/learning-about-down-syndrome
March of Dimes	Mission: improve the health of babies by preventing birth defects, premature birth, and infant mortality; includes health, stories research, and professional topics and information on birth defects and other health conditions	www.marchofdimes.org/complications/birth-defects-and-health-conditions.aspx

(continued)

TABLE 9.6 Selected Online Resources for Prenatal Genetic Risk Assessment (*continued*)		
Online Resource	Description	Weblink
National Society of Genetic Counselors	Health care provider site with information about genetic counselors; benefits of a genetic counselor and genetic counseling in practice	nsgc.org/p/cm/ld/fid=46
National Organization for Rare Diseases (NORD)	Tools and resources on rare diseases	rarediseases.org
Society for Maternal–Fetal Medicine	Information about maternal-fetal medicine specialization	www.smfm.org/what -is-the-society
Unique Chromosomal Disorder	International group supporting, informing, and networking with anyone affected by rare chromosome disorders and with any interested professionals	rarechromo.org/html/home.asp

(e.g., geneticist; prenatal genetic counselor; AGN). The process of inform-ing and supporting patients is often aided by online and written resources that can help the practitioner or be given to patients. Table 9.6 is a list of some of the many online resources providing information about medical genetic references, rare disorders, and issues related to prenatal care. Many centers have a collaborative team approach to prenatal care, includ-ing obstetricians, geneticist(s), genetic counselors, APRNs/nurse practitio-ners, and other specialized providers. Trained and certified AGNs often play a vital role in this process, by effective screening in order to identify the at-risk patient, preparing the patient and her significant others for the screening and testing process, and making important decisions and referrals.

> **Info Box**
>
> - The personal and family history is an integral part of the genetic assessment for preconception and prenatal care.
> - *Pre- and posttest genetic counseling* is part of the prenatal screening and diagnosis process and ethical, legal, and social implications (ELSI) must be considered as part of the process.

Summary

The risk-assessment process is important in preconception counseling and prenatal care. An important part of the process is a thorough personal and family history. Myriad screening and diagnostic tests are available to aid in the assessment process, depending on the individual's history and potential risks. APRNs should be knowledgeable as to how the risk-assessment process impacts maternal and fetal well-being and the potential for genetic conditions. Knowing resources for referral is central in communication and management of patients who are risk for genetic/genomic disorders.

References

Allen, J. F., Stoll, K., & Bernhardt, B. A. (2016). Pre- and post-test genetic counseling for chromosomal and Mendelian disorders. *Seminars in Perinatology, 40,* 44–55.

American College of Medical Genetics and Genomics. (2016, July 28). ACMG releases updated position statement on noninvasive prenatal screening (NIPS) for detection of fetal aneuploidy: Addresses questions about expanded roles of NIPS in prenatal practice. Retrieved from https://www.acmg.net/docs/NIPS_Final.pdf

American College of Obstetricians and Gynecologists. (2005 [reaffirmed 2015]). The importance of preconception care in the continuum of women's health care. *ACOG Committee Opinion.* Retrieved from http://www.acog.org/Resources-And-Publications/Committee -Opinions/Committee-on-Gynecologic-Practice/The-Importance-of-Preconception-Care-in-the -Continuum-of-Womens-Health-Care

American College of Obstetricians and Gynecologists. (2013, December). The use of chromosomal microarray analysis in prenatal diagnosis. Retrieved from https://www.acog.org/ About-ACOG/News-Room/News-Releases/2013/Ob-Gyns-Recommend-Chromosomal -Microarray-Analysis

American College of Obstetricians and Gynecologists. (2014, April). Screening tests for birth defects. Retrieved from http://www.acog.org/Patients/FAQs/Screening-Tests-for-Birth-Defects

American College of Obstetricians and Gynecologists. (2015a, September). Cell-free DNA screening for fetal aneuploidy. Retrieved from http://www.acog.org/Resources-And-Publications/ Committee-Opinions/Committee-on-Genetics/Cell-free-DNA-Screening-for-Fetal-Aneuploidy

American College of Obstetricians and Gynecologists. (2015b, September). Diagnostic tests for birth defects. Retrieved from https://www.acog.org/Patients/FAQs/Diagnostic-Tests-for-Birth -Defects

American College of Obstetricians and Gynecologists Committee on Genetics. (2017, March). Carrier screening for genetic conditions, Number 691. Retrieved from https://www.acog.org/ Resources-And-Publications/Committee-Opinions/Committee-on-Genetics/Carrier-Screening -for-Genetic-Conditions

Dey, M., Sharma, S., & Aggarwal, S. (2013). Prenatal screening methods for aneuplodies. *North American Journal of Medical Sciences*, *5*(3), 182–190.

Edwards, Q. T., Seibert, D., Macri, C., Covington, C., & Tilghman, J. (2004). Assessing ethnicity in preconception counseling: Genetics—What nurse practitioners need to know. *Journal of the American Academy of Nurse Practitioners*, *16*(11), 472–480.

Egan, J. F. (2004). Down syndrome births in the U.S. from 1989 to 2001. *American Journal of Obstetrics & Gynecology*, *191*(3), 1044–1048. Retrieved from https://commons.wikimedia.org/ wiki/File:Down_Syndrome_Risk_By_Age.png

Griffiths, A. J. F., Miller, J. H., Suzuki, D. E., Lewontin, R. C., & Gelbart, W. M. (2000). Aneuploidy. In *An introduction to genetic analysis* (7th ed.). New York, NY: W. H. Freeman. Retrieved from http://www.ncbi.nlm.nih.gov/books/NBK21870

Guraya, S. (2013). The associations of nuchal translucency and fetal abnormalities: Significance and implications. *Journal of Clinical and Diagnostic Research: JCDR*, *7*(5), 936–941. doi:10.7860/JCDR/2013/5888.2989

Hook, E. B., Cross, P. K., & Schreinemachers, D. M. (1983). Chrowmosomal abnormality rates at amniocentesis and in live-born infants. *Journal of the American Medical Association*, *249*(14), 2034–2038.

Kataguiri, M. R., Araujo, E., Bussamra, L. C. S., Nardozza, L. M. M., & Moron, A. F. (2014). Influence of second-trimester ultrasound markers for Down syndrome in pregnant women of advanced age. *Journal of Pregnancy*. Retrieved from https://www.hindawi.com/journals/jp /2014/7857830

Lister Hill National Center for Biomedical Communications, U.S. National Library of Medicine, National Institutes of Health, Department of Health & Human Services. (2017, June 20). Help me understand genetics: Genetic testing. Retrieved from https://ghr.nlm.nih.gov/primer/testing.pdf

National Coalition for Health Professional Education in Genetics. (2016). Non-invasive prenatal testing (NIPT) [Factsheet]. Retrieved from http://www.nchpeg.org/documents/nipt _factsheet_table072712.pdf

National Society of Genetic Counselors. (n.d.-a). About genetic counselors. Retrieved from http://www.nsgc.org/page/aboutgeneticcounselors

National Society of Genetic Counselors. (n.d.-b). Healthcare providers—Genetic counselors by specialty. Retrieved from http://nsgc.org/p/cm/ld/fid=49=prenatal

Nazareth, S. B., Lazarin, G. A., & Goldberg, J. D. (2015). Changing trends in carrier screening for genetic disease in the United States. *Prenatal Diagnosis, 35*(10), 931–935.

Newberger, D. (2000). Down syndrome: Prenatal risk assessment and diagnosis. *American Family Physician, 62*(4), 825–832, 837–838.

Norwitz, E. R., & Levy, B. (2013). Noninvasive prenatal testing: The future is now. *Reviews in Obstetrics and Gynecology, 6*(2), 48–62.

Nypayer, C., Arbour, M., & Niederegger, E. (2016). Preconception care: Improving the health of women and families. *Journal of Midwifery & Women's Health, 61*(3), 356–364.

Park, N. J., Morgan, C., Sharma, R., Li, Y., Lobo, R. M., Redman, J. B., . . . Strom, C. M. (2010). Improving accuracy of Tay–Sachs carrier screening of the non-Jewish population: Analysis of 34 carriers and six late-onset patients with HEXA enzyme and DNA sequence analysis. *Pediatric Research, 67*, 217–220.

Renna, M. D., Pisani, P., Conversano, F., Perrone, E., Casciaro, E., Di Renzo, G. C., . . . Casciaro, S. (2013). Sonographic markers for early diagnosis of fetal malformations. *World Journal of Radiology, 5*(10), 356–371.

Scott, S. A., Edelmann, L., Liu, L., Luo, M., Desnick, R. J., & Kornreich, R. (2010). Experience with carrier screening and prenatal diagnosis for sixteen Ashkenazi Jewish genetic disease. *Human Mutation, 31*(11), 1240–1250.

Society for Maternal-Fetal Medicine, Dugoff, L., Norton, M. E., & Kuller, J. A. (2016). The use of chromosomal microarray for prenatal diagnosis. *American Journal of Obstetrics & Gynecology, 215*(4), B2–B9. Retrieved from http://www.sciencedirect.com/science/article/pii/S0002937816304501

Souka, A. P., Von Kaisenberg, C. S., Hyett, J. A., Sonek, J. D., & Nicolaides, K. H. (2005). Increased nuchal translucency with normal karyotype. *American Journal of Obstetrics & Gynecology, 192*(4), 1005–1021.

Spaggiari, E., Czerkiewica, I., Sault, C., Dreux, S., Galland, A., Salomon, L. J., . . . Muller, F. (2016). Impact of including or removing nuchal translucency measurement on the detection and false-positive rates of first-trimester Down syndrome screening. *Fetal Diagnosis and Therapy, 40*(3), 214–218.

Thompson, A. E. (2015). Noninvasive prenatal screening. *Journal of the American Medical Association, 314*(2), 198. Retrieved from http://jama.jamanetwork.com/article.aspx?articleid=2396480

Wienke, S., Brown, K., Farmer, M., & Strange, C. (2014). Expanded carrier screening panels: Does bigger mean better? *Journal of Community Genetics, 5*(2), 191–198.

10

Newborns, Infants, and Children

Ann H. Maradiegue

Genomic risk assessment of the pediatric population includes the recognition of genetic disorders including physical and dysmorphology features that may be present in some disorders that are indicative of disease. Equally important is the monitoring of growth, development, and milestones of infants and children in order to identify disease. This requires not only a basic knowledge and understanding of genetics/genomics and patterns of inheritance, but also recognition of the normal physical and psychosocial patterns of growth and behavior that occur in the developing child. Additionally, ethical issues related to genetic testing can provide unique challenges in this age group.

Objectives

1. Discuss the skills required to conduct a genetic/genomic risk assessment for the pediatrics patient

2. Explain newborn screening (NBS)

3. Outline the genomic RISK assessment process for the pediatric patient

4. Discuss ethical, legal, and social issues related to genomic testing in the pediatric population

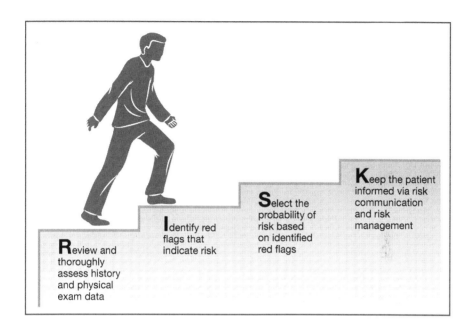

Newborn Screening

Preconception counseling is important in preparing individuals and couples for pregnancy and provides a means to begin assessment for potential maternal–fetal risk that may occur during pregnancy. Preconception counseling enables interventions to be employed to reduce risk (e.g., folic acid; smoking cessation) and carrier genetic testing to be offered based upon personal and family history to identify potential risk for genetic disease to the infant. During pregnancy, early and continuous prenatal care enables health care providers, including advanced practice registered nurses (APRNs), to continue the maternal/fetal risk assessment process through obtainment of a comprehensive personal and family history, physical examination, and implementation of ancillary tests (e.g., ultrasound; prenatal blood tests—maternal serum alpha-fetoprotein [MSAFP]). Chapter 9 provides information on the genetic/genomic risk assessment process during the preconception and prenatal period.

After delivery, assessment for genetic/genomic disorders continues through NBS. NBS "identifies conditions that can affect a child's long-term health or survival through early detection and diagnosis for the purpose of implementing interventions to prevent death or disability enabling children to reach their full potential" (Centers for Disease Control and Prevention [CDC], 2016b, para. 1). NBS was introduced to the United States in 1963 with the phenylalanine hydroxylase deficiency test, traditionally knows as phenylketonuria or PKU. Today, all 50 states screen newborns for PKU, galactosemia, and congenital hypothyroidism with additional routine newborn assessment for developmental, genetic, and metabolic disorders performed, with the type and number of tests varying by state. NBS also includes optoacoustic emissions (OAE) testing for hearing loss, allowing early identification and intervention for deafness and hearing impairment (National Human Genome Research Institute [NHGRI], 2016). Like other screening programs, NBS may generate false positive results. Babies who screen positive are referred to specialists for diagnostic testing and intervention if needed. More information about screening in different states is provided in Table 10.1.

Although the NBS tests provide a means to identify and diagnose a wide range of conditions in the newborn, it is not all inclusive and many other genetic or chromosomal disorders may exist warranting the need for risk assessment. The acronym RISK can be used in the risk assessment process regarding newborn assessment for genetic/genomic conditions.

Review of History

The maternal, paternal, and family history play a major role in assessment of genetic/genomic risk for numerous issues including single-gene disorders; chromosomal or polygenetic disorders; microdeletion syndromes; environmental issues (e.g., radiation exposures, teratogens); infectious diseases (e.g., Zika, toxoplasmosis, other agents, rubella, cytomegalovirus, herpes simplex [TORCH]); or occupational exposures (e.g., organic solvents). Of importance is the maternal history during the prenatal period: *What was the age of the mother at the time of delivery? Did the patient receive prenatal care? When was prenatal care initiated during the pregnancy? Was any prenatal screening or testing conducted? If prenatal tests were conducted, when were they conducted, what was performed, and what were the findings? Were there any abnormal prenatal tests?* In addition, a review of the mother's medical history (e.g., diabetes; hypertension), obstetric (OB) history (e.g., multiple miscarriages), and behavioral history to include smoking, prescription medication, over-the-counter (OTC) medications, and drug and alcohol use should be assessed as these

TABLE 10.1 Selected Online Resources for Newborn Screening

Online Resource	Description	Weblink
Centers for Disease Control and Prevention	Public health initiative to provide information and resources on newborn screening, resources, and tools	www.cdc.gov/ newbornscreening
Baby's First Test	Offers a series of guidelines, testing information by state, and resources for health professionals	www.babysfirsttest.org/ newborn-screening/health -professionals
March of Dimes	Information for parents about newborn screening and health tips	www.marchofdimes.org/ baby/newborn-screening -tests-for-your-baby.aspx
National Newborn Screening and Global Resource Center	Newborn screening information with additional facts about genetic disorders, testing, and fact sheets	genes-r-us.uthscsa.edu/ resources/consumer/statemap .htm
American College of Medical Genetics (ACMG)	Mission of ACMG is to develop and sustain genetic and genomic initiatives in clinical and laboratory practice, education, and advocacy	www.acmg.net/Search ?SearchTerms=newborn screening
U.S. Department of Health and Human Services	Advisory Committee on Heritable Disorders in Newborns and Children recommended uniform screening panel	www.hrsa.gov/ advisorycommittees/ mchbadvisory/ heritabledisorders/ recommendedpanel

(*continued*)

TABLE 10.1 Selected Online Resources for Newborn Screening (*continued*)		
Online Resource	Description	Weblink
American Academy of Pediatrics	Newborn screening website	https://www.aap.org/en-us/advocacy-and-policy/aap-health-initiatives/PEHDIC/pages/newborn-screening.aspx
Save Babies Through Screening Foundation	State-by-state view of newborn screening	www.savebabies.org/screening.html

factors can have an impact on the infant at the time of delivery and later in life. Specific information regarding the pregnancy (e.g., intrauterine growth retardation, placental morphology) and delivery history (e.g., bleeding, fetal distress), birth weight, and Apgar scores, as well as other pertinent data, should also be evaluated. Scores using the new Ballard system can provide an assessment of a newborn's gestational age (Phillips et al., 2013). Additional screening for hypoglycemia should be performed on newborns who are large or small for gestational age, or whose mothers were treated for gestational diabetes. Another important area that should always be explored with the family includes psychosocial situation (e.g., teenage or single mother, financial distress), as this has the potential to have long-term impacts on the newborn well into childhood.

The family history is also an important part of the genetic/genomic risk assessment. Any significant history on both the maternal and paternal lineages should be assessed regarding its significance to the health of the newborn. Ancestry of origin history may play an important role in identifying potential genetic disorders that are found at higher rates among certain racial/ethnic populations (e.g., Eastern Europeans, Ashkenazi Jews) and a history of consanguinity may increase the risk for autosomal recessive (AR) disorders. A review of the family history, including evaluation of the children's medical history (e.g., family history of birth defects, learning/mental disabilities, or genetic conditions), may also reveal conditions that may have a familial or inherited predisposition.

The physical examination of the newborn is central to the risk assessment process during the newborn period and continues to be an essential component of the assessment throughout pediatric development. The history data described previously in conjunction with the physical examination may reveal red flags that suggest a genetic or chromosomal disorder. Assessment of the newborn for features or characteristics that denote *dysmorphology*, "defined as the study of abnormal physical development" (Jorde, Carey, & Bamshad, 2016, p. 301), is an essential component of the physical exam. The newborn should have a thorough, systematic physical examination that includes weight, length, head circumference, and assessment of the skin, head and neck, heart and lungs, abdomen, genitalia, and nervous system, as well as reflexes to evaluate for abnormal development that may denote a genetic or medical condition. Similar examinations should occur throughout infancy and childhood. Of significance is the appearance of any abnormal characteristics or features that may be suggestive of a genetic/genomic condition warranting further evaluation or genetic testing. Infants who are born prematurely, with medical conditions, or have other problems may warrant additional assessment or tests. See Table 10.2 for components of a physical examination of the newborn, including examples of abnormalities that may be found based on the system.

Identification of Risk

Identification of risk is based on information obtained from the risk assessment process or screening tests. NBS tests are done within the first week of life to identify disorders before symptoms appear so that lifesaving interventions can be initiated. These screening tests help to identify potentially treatable or manageable congenital disorders within days of birth. Life-threatening health problems, mental disabilities, and serious lifelong disabilities can be avoided or minimized if a condition is quickly identified and treated. The tests are organized into broad categories: metabolic disorders (e.g., PKU, galactosemia); endocrine disorders (e.g., congenital hypothyroidism; congenital adrenal hyperplasia); hemoglobin disorders (e.g., sickle cell anemia); and other disorders (e.g., cystic fibrosis; American Association for Clinical Chemistry, n.d.; March of Dimes, 2016).

TABLE 10.2 Selected Components of a Newborn Physical Examination With Examples of Abnormalities

System	Examination	Examples of Abnormalities

Is there *observable malformation/anomaly* (e.g., cleft lip/palate; meningocele; absence of digits)? Is the malformation or anomaly associated with a genetic/chromosomal syndrome?

System	Examination	Examples of Abnormalities
Vital signs (normal levels)	• Heart rate 120–160 beats/min • Respiratory rate 40–60 breaths/min • Systolic blood pressure 60–90 mmHg • Temperature 97.7°F–99.5°F • Weight approximately 6–9 lb • Length 19–21 in. • Pulse oximetry ≥95%	Anything outside of the normal range (e.g., birth weight above the 90th percentile or greater than 9 lb)
Head	• Head circumference (normal range 13–15 in.) • Head shape • Fontanelles (anterior 3–6 cm, posterior 1–1.5 cm)	Microcephaly (indicates central nervous system malformation; Zika virus) Macrocephaly (hydrocephalus or brain tumor); prematurely fused skull (craniosynostosis) limits growth and 20% are associated with single-gene mutations
Eyes	• Eye color • Palpebral fissures (slanting) • Inner canthal distance • Pupil size • Appearance (of conjunctiva, sclera, and eyelid) • Red reflex • Assess corneal opacities	Genetic syndromes often cause unusual eye shapes, hyper/hypotelorism (Down syndrome, fetal alcohol syndrome, and colobomas) Abnormal red reflex warrants immediate referral Newborns with family history of retinoblastoma should be referred

(continued)

TABLE 10.2 Selected Components of a Newborn Physical Examination With Examples of Abnormalities (*continued*)

System	Examination	Examples of Abnormalities
Ears	• Size, shape, and position of ears • Hearing evaluation (otoacoustic emissions test) to take place before 1 month of age • There is a known association between ear and renal abnormalities	Low set ears are often a sign of a genetic condition (e.g., *Down, Turner, or trisomy 18*) Isolated ear anomalies: Preauricular pits or cup ears associated with dysmorphic features, teratogenic exposures, family history of deafness, or maternal history of gestational diabetes. (Any newborn with isolated auricular anomaly should have ultrasonography of kidneys.)
Nose	• Assess patency of both nostrils, asymmetry of nasal septum	Choanal atresia; encephalocele
Mouth	• Assess mouth, maxilla, mandible for fit and opening at equal angles, frenulum, and natal teeth	Cleft lip/palate most common anomalies of the head/ neck; short, long, or flat philtrum
Neck	• Inspect range of motion, webbing, clefts, pits, or fractures	Webbing can occur with *Turner syndrome*
Heart	• Assess pulses, murmurs (benign murmurs common in the first hours of life), cyanosis	Tricuspid atresia, transposition of the great arteries

(*continued*)

TABLE 10.2 Selected Components of a Newborn Physical Examination With Examples of Abnormalities (*continued*)

System	Examination	Examples of Abnormalities
Lungs	• Assess for respiratory distress (e.g., tachypnea, nasal flaring, grunting, retractions, cyanosis)	*Cystic fibrosis*, primary ciliary dyskinesia
Skin	• Color and integrity of skin and hair; birthmarks, erythema, milia, or pustules	Little or no pigmentation of skin and hair *albinism*
Chest	• Observe for symmetric movement, nipple placement, and any deformities (e.g., pectus carniatum and excavatum generally inconsequential)	Asymmetry suggests pneumothorax, wide nipple placement seen in Turner syndrome, prominent precordium may be seen in heart defect
Abdomen	• Observation for hernias or distension, omphalocele, bowel sounds, and organomegaly • Umbilical cord for signs of infection, number of arteries (two) and veins (one)	About one-half of the masses are renal in origin (e.g., Wilms tumor) A single umbilical artery is associated with other congenital malformations
Genitourinary	• Inspect for any abnormalities, and problems with urination	Ambiguous genitalia warrants evaluation by geneticist before gender assignment; hypospadias
Anus/rectum	• Examine for normal placement and patency, problems with defecation, dimples, hairy patches	Imperforate anus

(*continued*)

TABLE 10.2 Selected Components of a Newborn Physical Examination With Examples of Abnormalities (*continued*)		
System	Examination	Examples of Abnormalities
Extremities	• Inspect for abnormalities of hands, finger, feet, and toes • Evaluate for brachial plexus injury, hip dysplasia, talipes equinovarus, and pedal edema	Syndactyly, polydactyly; single palmar crease may be seen in trisomy 21 (Figure 10.1); pedal edema in the newborn may indicate *Turner syndrome*
Neuromuscular	Examination to elicit primitive instincts and muscle tone	Congenital myopathies

Note: Areas in italics suggest genetic or chromosomal abnormalities.
Sources: Lewis (2014a, 2014b).

Newborns with red flags based upon the maternal or familial history and/or the physical examination warrant further evaluation based upon the findings to determine if the history data and/or clinical features are suggestive of a genetic condition warranting genetic counseling and consideration for genetic testing. Referral for expert evaluation via a geneticist or pediatrician would be required for further evaluation.

Selecting Probability of Risk

Selecting probability of risk is based on the history, physical examination, and/or screening tests. Some physical characteristics have a high probability of a specific disorder that requires further evaluation for diagnosis. One example of a case history is as follows:

Sample Case

A 46-year-old, married, White female, gravida 1 para 1-0-0-1, of Northern European ancestry delivered a female infant at 40.3 weeks gestation via vaginal delivery; the patient had no prenatal care due to lack of insurance but delivered via hospitalization upon entering the emergency department with symptoms of labor; medical history is unremarkable; no use of medications including OTC; denies tobacco, alcohol, or illegal drug use; additional social and behavioral history is unremarkable; the third-generation family history revealed history of chronic conditions late in life among grandparents, otherwise family history was uneventful; infant: weight 8 lb. 3 oz., length 21 cm; physical examination of the newborn revealed noteworthy dysmorphic facial features with *upslanting palpebral fissures; small head, ears, and mouth, flattened facial profile of nose and maxillary region; short neck extremities with single, deep crease across the palm of the hand—simian crease* (Figure 10.1); and *hypotonia*. The clinical features revealed red flags that were strongly suggestive of a chromosomal disorder associated with Down syndrome. Further assessment and testing was conducted that revealed trisomy 21; the infant was later diagnosed with Down syndrome.

In the sample case, the infant had common physical features of Down syndrome that had a high probability of being diagnosed with the syndrome. Examples of common features of the disorder include flattened face, especially the nose; upslanting palpebral fissures or almond-shaped eyes; short neck; small ears; tongue that tends to stick out or protrude from

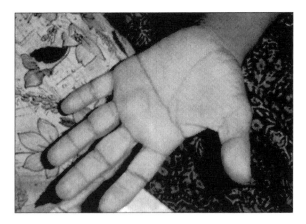

FIGURE 10.1 A depiction of an older child with a single palmar crease formerly known as a simian crease.

Source: Verma and Sodhi (2009).

the mouth; small hands and feet; single palmar crease (observable in approximately 50% of individuals); poor muscle tone or loose joints; shortened height; and small pinky finger (CDC, 2016a; Jorde et al., 2016).

Keep the Parent Up to Date

Newborns with a suspicious maternal or family history, and/or personal exam findings suggestive of Down or other syndromes, warrant further evaluation and diagnosis for the syndrome. Families are often devastated to find out that their expectations of a perfect child have not been fulfilled. The challenge is to establish, with the parents, the amount of information and support required for the child and for them to function. Care for families with a sick newborn is usually administered by a multidisciplinary team. Findings indicate that the best approach is to have a team well versed in the child's anomaly, who can discuss all the possible outcomes, and yet is realistic without taking away the family's hope; these are the skills that are most appreciated by the parents of a newborn with a disorder (Miguel-Verges et al., 2009). Depending upon the setting and expertise available at the institution, referrals may be required and support resources should be made available.

Although this book is unable to provide myriad genetic/genomic conditions that can occur in newborns or children, there are certain concepts that can further aid in evaluating birth defects. Of importance is that 10% to 15% of major congenital anomalies are due to single-gene defects and 5% to 10% due to chromosomal abnormalities or rearrangements with *most* due to unknown causality, multigenetic/nongenetic (polygenetic) factors, or environmental/nongenetic factors like that of exposure to infections or teratogens (Repetto, 2012, p. 26). Table 10.3 provides examples of commonly used concepts regarding birth defects.

It is important to know that some congenital malformations can be reduced or prevented through avoiding use of known teratogens (e.g., carbamazepine, valproic acid associated with neural tube defects), implementation of healthy lifestyles through avoidance of alcohol, and administration of folic acid as part of preconception counseling or use in early pregnancy. Ongoing review of history data prior to and during pregnancy is an important part of the risk assessment process so that primary and secondary prevention can be implemented to reduce the risk of many birth defects.

TABLE 10.3 Common Concepts Used in Describing Birth Defects (Not All Inclusive)	
Concept	Definition (Examples)
Approximately 2% to 3% of newborns have major congenital abnormalities[a]	

Malformation/anomaly
a. Malformation syndrome
b. Sequence
	Congenital morphological anomaly of a single organ or body part present at birth that can be caused by multiple factors such as genetic, prenatal events, unknown (e.g., cleft palate; anencephaly)
	    a. Pattern of multiple primary malformations that share a common etiology (e.g., Down syndrome)
	    b. Group of anomalies rising from an initial malformation

Association	Group of anomalies occurring together (e.g., vertebral defects, anal atresia, cardiac defects, tracheo-esophageal fistula, renal anomalies, and limb abnormalities [VACTERL/VATER])[b]
Dysplasia	Morphologic abnormality resulting in organ, tissue, or structural changes (e.g., achondroplasia)[c]

Sources: [a]Repetto (2012); [b]Solomon (2011); [c]Jorde et al. (2016).

Pediatrics

Review of Data

Review of data in pediatrics is continued as the child develops to ensure the health and safety of the child. The personal and family history is updated during every visit to identify any changes in the health of family members and any complications (e.g., recent illnesses or deaths). Pediatrics in the primary care setting requires the skills to monitor, evaluate, and refer to specialists for genetic/genomic illnesses throughout the stages of growth and development.

Identification of Genetic RISK

Identification of genetic risk in pediatric patients deals with disorders not previously identified through NBS or the newborn exam. Pediatric conditions that are considered red flags include intellectual disabilities, congenital hearing loss, and family members with diseases that will affect the child later in life. Additionally, there are many tests available to assist with identification of genetic disorders.

The development of chromosome analysis, starting in 1959 with the recognition of trisomy 21, rapidly increased the ability to determine the etiology of many birth defects. Chromosome abnormalities represent 5% to 10% of birth defects. Although most common chromosome abnormalities are well known (e.g., trisomies 21, 13, and 18, Turner syndrome, and Klinefelter syndrome), many are seen less frequently and are less well known, like that of the sex chromosome abnormalities, XXX and XYY. Even more striking is the fact that structural chromosome abnormalities (e.g., deletions, duplications, translocations, and inversions), although they can be familial, are typically unique and sporadic. This can make it difficult to predict the prognosis, making the diagnosis hard to comprehend (O'Connor, 2008).

With the advent of DNA analysis, newer methods of laboratory analysis have been developed. Fluorescent in situ hybridization (FISH) enabled us to tag specific genes with fluorescent markers that could be seen under the microscope. Gene sequencing enabled identification of sequence variations leading to disease. Then in 2004, genetic diagnosis was revolutionized with the introduction of chromosome microarray analysis. More recently, whole genome sequencing (WGS) and whole exome sequencing (WES) are opening a whole new method of laboratory assessment, allowing diagnosis not previously possible. Table 10.4 summarizes the different genetic testing methods available. Although classic genetic testing has long been used in the identification of single-gene disorders, genomics is showing us a wide array of changes that affect gene expression. For example, changes in methylation and differential gene expression can result in Prader–Willi syndrome, dependent upon which parental gene is expressed (Driscoll, Miller, Schwartz, & Cassidy, 1998/2016).

Selecting Probability of Risk

Selecting probability of risk is dependent upon the disorder. Although new tools and techniques have provided important diagnostic

TABLE 10.4 Selected Genetic Tests Used in Pediatrics

Test	Description	Applications
Biochemical assays	Many types available, depending on the condition	Some can be performed only on certain tissue types, and only by specialized laboratories[a] The selection of the type of assay is critical; therefore, a biochemical workup is often best directed by a subspecialist in inborn errors of metabolism[a]
FISH (fluorescence in situ hybridization) testing	Microscope-based study of a specific chromosomal region	FISH testing is used in many situations, but is now often replaced with microarray[a]
Karyotype	Microscope-based study of chromosomes	Used in many situations, including prenatally, in cancer genetics, and in patients with neurocognitive impairment and/or congenital malformations; in many situations, karyotyping is being replaced by microarray[a]
Microarray	Study of overall genomic material	Contains similar information to karyotyping, but is analyzed through different technology, and at much higher resolution[a]
Sequencing	Base-by-base examination of a portion of genetic material	Traditionally, a single gene or small group of genes would be sequenced if a mutation affecting that gene was suspected; however, new technologies now make simultaneous large-scale sequencing of many genes or the whole genome (WGS/WES) possible[b] *Note:* Certain specific diseases/anomalies (e.g., cardiac) may also be tested using a multigene or expanded gene panels

WES, whole exome sequencing; WGS, whole genome sequencing.

Sources: [a]Genetic Alliance; the New York–Mid-Atlantic Consortium for Genetic and Newborn Screening Services (2009); [b]Ng and Kirkness (2010).

breakthroughs, approximately 30% to 50% of the etiology of birth defects still remain unknown (Repetto, 2012). Therefore, it is important to conduct a good assessment focusing on personal and family history and physical examination, utilizing information from prior tests if conducted, evaluating any abnormal lab data, and observing for dysmorphology. Any unusual findings could indicate the *probability* of a genetic disorder warranting referral and further evaluation.

Observing for dysmorphic features is important in the pediatric assessment, particularly as it relates to genetics/genomics. A primary resource, *Smith's Recognizable Patterns of Human Malformation* (Jones, Jones, & del Campo, 2013), now in its seventh edition, stands as a major tool in physical recognition of genetic syndromes in the years leading up to the DNA age. This book aides the practitioner in making the genetic

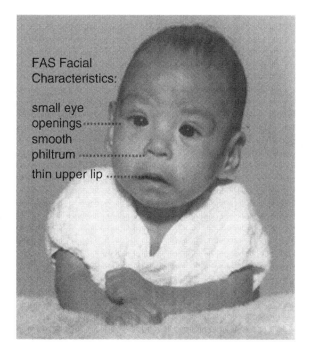

FIGURE 10.2 Fetal alcohol syndrome (FAS) with unique facial characteristics of this syndrome.

Source: commons.wikimedia.org/wiki/File:Photo_of_baby_with_FAS.jpg

diagnosis in the child with abnormalities. A few examples of malformations include cleft lip and palate, spina bifida, webbed neck as seen in Turner syndrome, disproportionally long legs and hands, arms and fingers as seen in Marfan syndrome, bulging eyes with telangiectasis and redundant skin folds of Ehlers–Danlos syndrome, and the characteristic facial features of fetal alcohol syndrome (Figure 10.2). There are also several dysmorphology databases available that require a subscription (e.g., POSSUM). Additional resources regarding pediatric genetic disorders are presented in Table 10.5.

TABLE 10.5 Selected Online Resources for Clinical Genetics for Pediatrics		
Online Resource	Description	Weblink
American Academy of Family Physicians	2014 Screening recommendations for sickle cell disease from expert panel	www.aafp.org/afp/ 2015/1215/p1069 .html
American Academy of Family Physicians	Care of children with Down syndrome	www.aafp.org/afp/ 2014/1215/p851.html
Genetics Home Reference	Provides many resources, including descriptions of conditions	ghr.nlm.nih.gov
National Human Genome Research Institute	A source for standardized terminology with links to articles	elementsofmorphology .nih.gov
National Organization of Rare Disorders	Patient-centered website with links to support groups and physicians that specialize in specific disorders	rarediseases.org
Unique	Information for families and providers on rare chromosome disorders	www.rarechromo.org/ html/home.asp

Currently, there is limited use of WGS/WES in children; these sequencing techniques are being used to assist with the diagnosis of children with undiagnosed rare disorders that warrant further evaluation and genetic evaluation. Although the use of these testing techniques is in its initial stage, WGS has the potential to identify any form of genetic variation, and WES has current usage for neurologic disorders and some congenital anomalies examining known coding regions for sequence mutations. In pediatric practice, genetic testing is often used for an existing clinical diagnosis or as part of a differential diagnosis, thereby establishing or ruling out a particular finding (Stavropoulos et al., 2016). The challenge in WGS/WES technology is in disclosure of the sequencing results and interpretation of these results as well as any unexpected findings including variants of unknown significance (VUS). What has been ascertained from the new sequencing techniques is that the relationship between genotype and phenotype is not always straightforward, meaning the distinction between diagnosis and risk assessment is not always clear. New technologies may also identify future disabilities that may or may not be preventable and will not become apparent until adulthood (Feero & Guttmacher, 2014).

Keep the Parent Up to Date

The focus of ethical, legal, and social implication (ELSI) guidelines in the pediatric population considers what is in the best interest of the child and the navigation of family perspectives that was endorsed by the American Academy of Pediatrics in 2013. The parents are in the position to consent for their children, requiring that they have all of the salient information to make decisions for genomic sequencing and understanding the complexity, broad scope, and consequences of the technology. Current ELSI considerations include how to address the following issues:

1. Diagnosis, regardless of whether or not the disease is treatable, along with the biopsychosocial consequences of the patient and parent/caregivers.

2. Risk assessment for future health to include early-onset conditions, diseases, or disabilities when the risk is modifiable. This can especially have far-reaching effects when there are serious, far-reaching consequences if measures are not taken to intervene.

3. Risk assessment for future health, later onset conditions, diseases, or disabilities, the risk of which is modifiable during childhood. The child's long-term health interests are protected and promoted to prevent adult onset conditions, diseases, or disabilities for which protective interventions can be initiated during childhood.

4. Pharmacogenomic results with immediate clinical application

5. Incidental or secondary findings of life-threatening conditions (McCullough et al., 2015)

The RISK assessment mnemonic provides guidance through the ongoing process of evaluation. Using the mnemonic as a guide, responsibilities when caring for the pediatric population include:

R (Review histories—personal, family, environment)
- Family history with a minimum of a three-generation pedigree
  - To identify individuals and other family members who will benefit from genetic services
- Birth history and any pregnancy complications
  - Certain health conditions (e.g., diabetes), pregnancy complications (e.g., eclampsia and/or infections), environmental toxins (e.g., lead), and lifestyle behaviors (e.g., smoking and alcohol use) can herald health problems for the child
- Comprehensive physical exams
  - Recognize physical features that require further exploration or are consistent with the diagnosis of a genetic disorder

I (Identify red flags)
- Note any information in the pedigree or history that is a red flag
  - Multiple miscarriages, maternal health problems, or siblings with health problems
- Recognize/address psychosocial issues (e.g., maternal depression)

S (Select risk probability[ties] if available—using evidence-based models)
- Documentation of pediatric milestones
  - Regular screening of physical and cognitive development in order to recognize early delays that may require further

interventions. Milestones should be consistent with age. Most developmental disabilities occur before birth, but can occur after birth due to injury, infection, and other factors. Low birth weight, multiple births, and premature births have all been associated with developmental delays (see Table 10.6 for developmental red flags).

K (Keep informed—through risk communication and management)
- Effective communication with parents and other health professions
- Collaboration with other health professionals
- Referrals to genetic specialists as indicated (American Academy of Pediatrics, 2016)

TABLE 10.6 Clinical Signs Suggestive of Developmental Red Flags

Development Delay From Birth to 24 Months

Birth to 3 months
- Rolling prior to 3 months
  - Evaluate for hypertonia
- Persistent fisting at 3 months
  - Evaluate for neuromotor dysfunction
- Failure to alert to environmental stimuli
  - Evaluate for sensory impairment

4 to 6 months
- Poor head control
  - Evaluate for hypotonia
- Failure to reach for objects by 5 months
  - Evaluate for motor, visual, or cognitive deficits
- Absent smile
  - Evaluate for visual loss
  - Evaluate for attachment problems
  - Is there a need to evaluate for maternal major depression?
  - Is there a need to consider child abuse or child neglect?

(continued)

TABLE 10.6 Clinical Signs Suggestive of Developmental Red Flags (*continued*)

Development Delay From Birth to 24 Months

6 to 12 months
- Persistence of primitive reflexes after 6 months
  - Evaluate for neuromuscular disorder
- Absent babbling by 6 months
  - Evaluate for hearing deficit
- Absent stranger anxiety by 7 months
  - May be related to multiple care providers
- W-sitting and bunny hopping at 7 months
  - Evaluate for adductor spasticity or hypotonia
- Inability to localize sound by 10 months
  - Evaluate for unilateral hearing loss
- Persistent mouthing of objects at 12 months
  - May indicate lack of intellectual curiosity

12 to 24 months
- Lack of consonant production by 15 months
  - Evaluate for mild hearing loss
- Lack of imitation by 16 months
  - Evaluate for hearing deficit
  - Evaluate for cognitive or socialization deficit
- Lack of protodeclarative pointing by 18 months
  - Problem in social relatedness
- Hand dominance prior to 18 months
  - May indicate contralateral weakness with hemiparesis
- Inability to walk up and down stairs at 24 months
  - May lack opportunity rather than motor deficit
- Persistent poor transitions in 21–24 months
  - May indicate pervasive developmental disorder
- Advanced noncommunicative speech (e.g., echolalia)
- Simple commands not understood suggest abnormality
  - Evaluate for autism
  - Evaluate for pervasive developmental disorder
- Delayed language development
  - Requires hearing loss evaluation in all children

Note: These findings do not necessarily indicate a genetic condition but may be associated with multifactorial, behavioral/social, or other complex issues. W-sitting is when a child is sitting on his or her bottom with both knees bent and the legs turned out away from the body. There are orthopedic and neurological developmental concerns.

Info Box

Disorders Associated With Developmental Delays

- Hearing loss—This can be an inherited disorder, or associated with infection during pregnancy such as cytomegalovirus, or head trauma
- Intellectual disability—This can be due to fragile X syndrome, fetal alcohol syndrome, or infections during pregnancy such as toxoplasmosis
- Autism spectrum disorder—Children who have a sibling with autism are at higher risk of also having the disorder
- Chromosomal abnormalities—Down syndrome, Turner syndrome

Source: CDC (2016c).

Summary

Risk assessment is an important tool to use in for the assessment of the pediatric patient in clinical practice. APRNs specializing in the care of infants and children should have the knowledge and skills to recognize red flags that may be suggestive of a genetic disorder or syndrome. Risk communication and management are crucial skills, as these APRNs must interface with parents and specialists to make important health decisions. Because of the continuous advances in the field of genetics, APRNs must keep abreast of issues relating to genetics/genomics including that of WGS and WES so that appropriate ethical issues and the interest of the child can be maintained. Table 10.5 provides additional educational resources for the APRNs pertaining to clinical pediatric genetics.

References

American Academy of Pediatrics. (2016). Genetics counseling. Retrieved from https://geneticsinprimarycare.aap.org/YourPractice/When-to-Refer/Pages/Genetic-Counseling.aspx

American Association for Clinical Chemistry. (n.d.). Screening tests for newborns. Retrieved from https://labtestsonline.org/understanding/wellness/a-newborn-1/a-newborn-2

Centers for Disease Control and Prevention. (2016a, March 3). Facts about Down syndrome. Retrieved from https://www.cdc.gov/ncbddd/birthdefects/downsyndrome.html

Centers for Disease Control and Prevention. (2016b, August 2). Newborn screening portal. Retrieved from https://www.cdc.gov/newbornscreening

Centers for Disease Control and Prevention. (2016c, August 31). Facts about developmental disabilities. Retrieved from https://www.cdc.gov/ncbddd/developmentaldisabilities/facts.html

Driscoll, D., Miller, J., Schwartz, S., & Cassidy, S. (1998 [updated 2016, February 4]). Prader-Willi syndrome. In R. A. Pagon, M. P. Adam, H. H. Ardinger, S. E. Wallace, A. Amemiya, L. J. H. Bean., . . . K. Stevens (Eds.), *GeneReviews*. Seattle: University of Washington. Retrieved from https://www.ncbi.nlm.nih.gov/books/NBK1330

Feero, W. G., & Guttmacher, A. E. (2014). Genomics, personalized medicine, and pediatrics. *Academic Pediatrics, 14*(1), 14–22. doi:10.1016/j.acap.2013.06.008

Genetic Alliance; the New York–Mid-Atlantic Consortium for Genetic and Newborn Screening Services. (2009, July 8). *Understanding genetics: A New York, Mid-Atlantic guide for patients and health professionals*. Washington, DC: Genetic Alliance. Retrieved from https://www.ncbi .nlm.nih.gov/books/NBK115563

Jones, K. L., Jones, M. C., & del Campo, M. (2013). *Smith's recognizable patterns of human malformation* (7th ed.). Philadelphia, PA: Elsevier.

Jorde, L. B., Carey, J. C., & Bamshad, M. J. (2016). *Medical genetics* (5th ed.). Philadelphia, PA: Elsevier.

Lewis, M. L. (2014a, September). A comprehensive newborn examination: Part I. General, head and neck, cardiopulmonary. *American Family Physician, 90*(5), 289–296.

Lewis, M. L. (2014b, September). A comprehensive newborn examination: Part II. Skin, trunk, extremities, neurologic. *American Family Physician, 90*(5), 297–302.

March of Dimes. (2016). Newborn screening tests for your baby. Retrieved from http://www .marchofdimes.org/baby/newborn-screening-tests-for-your-baby.aspx

McCullough, L., Brothers, K., Chung, W., Joffe, S., Koenig, B., Wilfond, B., & Yu, J. (2015). Professionally responsible disclosure of genomic sequencing results in pediatrics. *Pediatrics, 136*(4), e974–e982.

Miguel-Verges, F., Woods, L., Aucott, A., Boss, R., Sulpar, L., & Donohue, P. (2009, October). Prenatal consultation with a neonatologist for congenital anomalies: Parental perceptions. *Pediatrics, 124*(4), e573–e579. doi:10.1542/peds.2008-2865

National Human Genome Research Institute. (2016, May 11). Newborn screening. Retrieved from https://www.genome.gov/27556918/newborn-screening-fact-sheet

Ng, P., & Kirkness, E. (2010). Whole genome sequencing. *Methods in Molecular Biology, 628*, 215–226.

O'Connor, C. (2008). Chromosomal abnormalities: Aneuploidies. *Nature Education*, 1(1), 172.

Phillips, R. M., Goldstein, M., Houghland, K., Nandyal, R., Pizzica, A., Santa-Donato, A., . . . Yost, E. (2013). Multidisciplinary guidelines for the care of late preterm infants. *Journal of Perinatology*, 33(Suppl. 2), S5–S22.

Repetto, G. M. (2012). Congenital malformation syndromes. In A. Y. Elzouki, H. A. Harfi, H. M. Nazer, F. B. Stapleton, W. Oh, & R. J. Whitley (Eds.), *Textbook of clinical pediatrics* (Vol. 1, 2nd ed.). Heidelberg, Germany: Springer-Verlag.

Solomon, B. D. (2011). VACTERL/VATER Association. *Orphanet Journal of Rare Diseases*, 6(56). Retrieved from https://ojrd.biomedcentral.com/articles/10.1186/1750-1172-6-56

Stavropoulos, D. J., Merico, D., Jobling, R., Bowdin, S., Monfared, N., Thiruvahindrapuram, B., . . . Marshall, C. (2016). Whole-genome sequencing expands diagnostic utility and improves clinical management in paediatric medicine. *Genome Medicine*, 1. Retrieved from http://www.nature.com/articles/npjgenmed201512

Verma, S. K., & Sodhi, R. (2009). Down's syndrome and cardiac tamponade with pulmonary tuberculosis in adults. *Indian Journal of Human Genetics*, 15(2), 72–74.

11

Cancer and RISK Assessment

It is estimated that approximately 5% to 10% of cancers are inherited as a result of germline mutations. Inherited cancer syndromes result in an increased risk of a specific type of cancer as well as other cancers or conditions. This chapter focuses on hereditary cancer syndromes associated with breast and colon cancers. Like that of other genetic conditions, the importance of risk assessment is key to early recognition of the syndromes so that appropriate management of risk can be implemented, which includes enhanced surveillance, chemoprevention, or risk-reduction surgery, if applicable.

Objectives

1. Discuss the RISK assessment process when evaluating individuals for inherited breast cancer syndromes

2. Discuss the RISK assessment process when evaluating individuals for inherited colon cancer syndromes

3. Identify resources for risk communication and risk management when suspecting individuals for inherited cancer syndromes

Breast Cancer and Hereditary Breast Cancer Syndromes

Breast cancer is the most common form of cancer in women. Approximately one in eight women in the United States, or 12%, will develop invasive

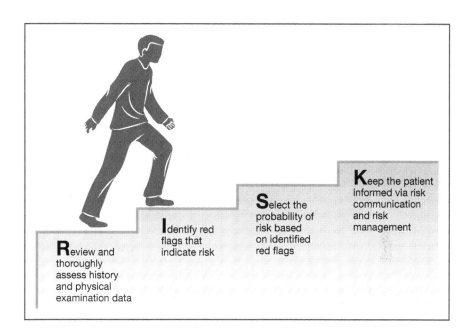

breast cancer during their lifetime (American Cancer Society [ACS], 2017e; Siegel, Miller, & Jamal, 2017). A myriad of nonmodifiable and modifiable factors are associated with breast cancer, and assessment of these factors play an important role in the risk assessment process and in identifying potential factors that may be suspect or red flags for inherited breast cancer syndromes. Table 11.1 includes examples of factors that can impact breast cancer risks.

Breast cancer risk assessment is important in identifying potential red flags that can be suspect for an inherited breast cancer syndrome. There are many types of breast cancer syndromes resulting from different pathogenic germline mutations, but the most common inherited form of the disease is that of hereditary breast and ovarian cancer (HBOC) syndrome due to mutations in the *BRCA1* or *BRCA2* genes (Lynch et al., 2007). Approximately 95% of families with inherited breast/ovarian cancer is due to mutation in *BRCA* (Ford et al., 1998). Although the syndrome is associated with increased lifetime (age 70) risk of breast (40%—80%) and ovarian cancer (15%–40% depending on the gene), there are other cancers and conditions that may occur as a result of the genetic mutation (Table 11.2; Petrucelli, Daly, & Feldman, 1998/2016). Even though HBOC makes up most of the hereditary breast cancer syndromes, there are other

TABLE 11.1 Breast Cancer Risk Factors

- *Noninherited/no history of germline mutation—nonmodifiable*
  - Increasing age (age 55 and older)
  - Gender (women 1:8 lifetime risk; men 1:1,000 lifetime risk[a])
  - Race/ethnicity
    - Caucasian high incidence; African Americans higher mortality rates and higher rates of age younger than 45 years
    - Increased incidence of *BRCA1* and *BRCA2* mutations among Ashkenazi Jews
  - Reproductive history
    - Early age of menarche (before age 12)
    - Nulliparity
    - Older age at first live birth
    - Older age at menopause (e.g., after age 55)
  - *Family history* (e.g., ~twofold risk with a first-degree relative [mother, sibling, daughter]; threefold increase with two first-degree relatives)
    - *Approximately 15% to 20% of breast cancers are familial[b]*
  - Breast density (mammography)
  - Breast lesions (examples)
    - Atypical ductal hyperplasia (ADH)[c]—four- to fivefold increase in risk (RR)
    - Atypical lobular hyperplasia (ALH)[c]—four- to fivefold increase in risk (RR)
    - Lobular carcinoma-in situ (LCIS)—tenfold increase in risk
  - Mantel radiation to the chest (children/young adults for certain cancers, Hodgkin's disease or non-Hodgkin's lymphoma) (e.g., prior thoracic radiation less than 30 years of age)

- *Noninherited modifiable*
  - Increased body mass index after menopause
  - Alcohol consumption (e.g., two- to fivefold increase in risk compared to 1.5-fold in those not using alcohol)
  - Physical inactivity
  - Current or prior estrogen and progesterone hormone therapy

- *Decreasing risk factors*
  - Breastfeeding
  - Prior oophorectomy before age 45 years
  - Physical activity
  - Prior risk-reducing therapy/surgery

RR, relative risk.

Sources: ACS, 2016; National Comprehensive Cancer Network (NCCN, 2016a); ACS 2017e; [b]Lynch, Silva, Snyder, and Lynch (2007); [c]Hartman, Degnim, Santen, Dupont, and Ghosh (2015).

TABLE 11.2 Inherited Syndromes Associated With Breast and/or Ovarian Cancer, and the Gene Mutation and Conditions and Cancers Associated With the Syndrome

Cancer Syndrome and (Inheritance Pattern)	Gene Mutation	Breast and Ovarian Cancer Risk and Other Conditions Associated With the Syndrome
Hereditary breast and ovarian cancer (AD)[a]	BRCA1 BRCA2	Breast (40%–80%); increased male breast cancer risk; Ovarian (15%–40%); peritoneal; fallopian tubes; melanoma; pancreatic; prostate
Partner and localizer of the BRCA2 gene[b] (AD)	PALB2	Breast (14%–35%); pancreatic cancer
Cowden syndrome[c] (AD)	PTEN	Breast (85% risk); endometrial cancer; follicular thyroid cancer (rarely papillary); gastrointestinal hamartomas; Lhermitte–Duclos disease (adult); skin changes (e.g., trichilemmomas; acral keratosis; oral papillomas; penile freckling; mucocutaneous neuromas; uterine fibroids; thyroid nodules/multinodular; macrocephaly
Li Fraumeni[d] (AD)	P53	Breast, particularly early age onset (50%); sarcoma (e.g., osteosarcoma; soft-tissue sarcomas); leukemia; central nervous system (brain); adrenocortical
Peutz–Jeghers[e] (AD)	STK11	Breast cancer (45%–50%); Ovarian (18%–21%); cancers: colorectal, gastric, pancreatic; Adenoma malignum of the cervix; benign neoplasm of ovary; Peutz–Jeghers type—hamartomatous polyps: small intestine; stomach; large bowel; mucotaneous macules predominantly in childhood

(*continued*)

TABLE 11.2 Inherited Syndromes Associated With Breast and/or Ovarian Cancer, and the Gene Mutation and Conditions and Cancers Associated With the Syndrome (continued)

Cancer Syndrome and (Inheritance Pattern)	Gene Mutation	Breast and Ovarian Cancer Risk and Other Conditions Associated With the Syndrome
Hereditary diffuse gastric cancer (AD)[f]	CDH1	Breast cancer (39%–52% lobular breast cancer); diffuse gastric cancer
Lynch syndrome[g] (AD)	MLH1 MSH2 MSH6 PMS2 EPCAM	Ovarian cancer (4%–24%); cancers: colon; endometrial; stomach; urinary (renal pelvis); brain; pancreas; hepatobiliary; sebaceous neoplasma
Ataxia-telangiectasia (AR)[h]	ATM	Breast cancer (28%); progressive cerebellar ataxia; telangiectasias; increased risk leukemia and lymphoma; sensitivity to ionizing radiation
Checkpoint kinase 2[i] (AD)	CHEK2	Breast (~20%–25%) increased colon, prostate

AD, autosomal dominant; AR, autosomal recessive.

Sources: [a]Petrucelli et al. (1998/2016); [b]Antoniou et al. (2014); [c]Eng (2016); [d]Mai et al. (2016); [e]McGarrity, Amos, and Baker (2001/2016); [f]Kaurah and Huntsman (2002/2014); [g]National Comprehensive Cancer Network (2017b); [h]Cybulski et al. (2011); [i]Lee et al. (2016).

inherited disorders associated with breast and ovarian cancer that must be considered when assessing individuals for an inherited cancer syndrome. Therefore, it is important that when assessing individuals for familial risk of breast cancer, particularly due to genetic mutations, a comprehensive personal and family history including physical examination should be conducted to assess for red flags that may be attributed to HBOC or other inherited cancer syndromes that increase the risk of breast and/or ovarian cancers. Table 11.2 presents a list of breast cancer syndromes caused by germline mutations including the gene associated as well as other conditions/cancers associated with the syndrome.

Although Table 11.2 presents a myriad of genes associated with inherited breast cancer, it is not all inclusive. Additional genes not shown in the table but associated with breast cancer include mutations in the *BRIP, NBN,* and *RAD50, RAD51C, RAD51D,* and *MRE11,* as well as other genes that are considered moderate penetrant genes (Kleibl & Kristensen, 2016; Mahdi, Nassin, & Nasin, 2013; NCI, 2017c; Ramus et al., 2015). Because of the various genes associated with breast and/or ovarian cancer, it is essential that advanced practice registered nurses (APRNs) without appropriate training *refer* patients suspect for an inherited breast cancer syndrome to an expert for appropriate genetic counseling and determination for genetic testing.

Review of History

The personal and family history is essential in determining familial and inherited (germline mutations) breast cancer risk. Important elements of the personal as well as family history are presented as each relates to the genomic risk assessment process when assessing for an inherited breast cancer syndrome.

Personal History

Current age of the proband/consultand should be obtained, including prior history of cancers and the age of onset of disease occurrence, pathology report(s), and treatment(s) given. Detailed medical and surgical history should also be obtained, including reproductive history (e.g., menstrual history; age of first birth; menopausal history) and prior surgical history, including breast biopsies and gynecological surgeries with pathology reports, as well as an annotation if prior surgery was conducted as a measure of risk-reduction, if applicable. Inquiry on the medication history, especially birth control and hormone use, should be included in the history data. Radiation exposures should also be assessed as this can increase cancer risks, including breast cancer. For instance, individuals exposed to mantel radiation for treatment of childhood cancers (e.g., Hodgkin's lymphoma) have up to a 40% increased risk of breast cancer by age 50 years (Moskowitz et al., 2014).

A focused physical exam should be conducted as part of the assessment; this includes breast, abdominal, and pelvic exams as well as evaluation of the *thyroid, head circumference, skin,* and *oral mucosa* due to Cowden syndrome, an inherited breast cancer syndrome that can manifest with macrocephaly (occipital frontal circumference ≥97th percentile or

≥58 cm for adult women and 60 cm for adult men; Shiovitz et al., 2010), and with dermatological characteristics and thyroid nodules (Eng, 2016; NCCN, 2017b; Table 11.2).

Family History

Check for patterns of inheritance and consanguinity on both the maternal and paternal lineages. A minimum three-generation pedigree is recommended as part of the assessment process. Always inquire about information on the ancestry of origin as some racial/ethnic groups are at higher risk for inherited breast cancer syndromes. For example, the frequency rate of *BRCA* mutations among individuals of Ashkenazi Jewish ancestry is one in 40 or 2.3%, compared to one in 500 or 0.2% for the general population; these rates further increase based on age and family history (Hartge, Struewing, Wacholder, Brody, & Tucker, 1999). In addition, three founder mutations—*BRCA1* (185delAG or 5382insC) and *BRCA2* (6174delT)— have been shown to occur frequently in the Ashkenazi Jewish population among those with HBOC (Hartge et al., 1999; Streuwing et al., 1997). Another part of the family history is to observe the family structure in the history data or depicted on the pedigree that may limit patterns of inheritance due to early-age onset of death for some members, paternal inheritance with few to no females on the paternal lineage, or adoption (see Figures 7.1 and 7.2). Current age of family members; pertinent medical/ surgical history, particularly cancer history and age of onset of disease; type of cancers; bilaterality; chemoprevention; and risk-reduction surgery should also be assessed, documented, and reviewed as it pertains to family members (NCCN, 2017b).

Identify Red Flags

There are personal, familial, and clinical manifestations that are considered red flags for hereditary breast cancer syndromes. Table 11.3 provides examples of some elements of risk that are considered red flags for possible inherited breast cancer syndromes, warranting APRNs to consider the need for further follow-up.

Select a Risk Probability

If identified red flags are present, discuss with the patient genetic referral for counseling, further evaluation, and possible genetic testing. If needed,

TABLE 11.3 Red Flags That May Be Suspect for a Familial or Inherited Breast Cancer Risk

- Early age onset of breast cancer in proband or family member
- Male breast cancer (personal or family history)
- Multiple family members with breast cancer
- One or more close family member (first, second, or third degree) with ovarian/fallopian tube or primary peritoneal cancer at any age
- Personal history of ovarian cancer
- Triple negative breast cancer diagnosis (estrogen, progestin, and HER2 negative) at age 60 or younger
- Known family member with a germline mutation for an inherited cancer syndrome
- High-risk/at-risk groups/populations based on ancestry of origin (e.g., Ashkenazi Jewish ancestry), particularly with a history of breast, ovarian, or pancreatic cancer
- Cancer or medical history in the proband or family members suspect for other inherited cancer syndrome (e.g., macrocephaly and Cowden syndrome or clinical manifestations)

HER2, human epidermal growth factor receptor 2.
Sources: ACS (2016); NCCN (2016a, 2017b).

have the patient procure personal pathology reports and medical records as well as death certificates, if needed, of cancer, medical disorders, or cause of death is uncertain or ambiguous and/or the family member's diagnosis of cancer warrants confirmation. Individuals with a known gene mutation in the family are considered at high risk for breast cancer until genetic testing has been conducted and reveals *no mutation found* for the mutated gene; this would constitute a true negative finding.

Individuals without a personal or family history of risk factors, including no behavioral/lifestyle or environmental risks, are considered at population or *average risk*. The population risk for breast cancer is approximately 12%, or one in eight for women and one in 1,000 for men.

Keep Individuals Informed

Keep the individuals informed of findings through risk communication and risk management.

Risk Communication and Management

Individuals without a personal or family history suggestive of breast cancer risk or without any personal or family history of red flags are at *average/population breast cancer risk* and should be counseled on appropriate breast cancer screening based on age unless determined otherwise. Primary preventive measures to further reduce risk should also be a part of risk communication and management and include regular exercise, reducing alcohol consumption if applicable, and maintaining a healthy weight. *Breast cancer risk estimate* based on age, personal reproductive history, and family history can also be evaluated using an empiric risk model like that of the Gail model. This model may be useful in determining the need for chemoprevention counseling. Other models are also available to determine the empiric risk for breast cancer (e.g., Claus model; Tyrer-Cuzick model).

Individuals with an *above-average breast cancer risk,* but whose personal and/or family history is *thoroughly assessed* and NOT *suggestive of an inherited syndrome* because of lack of red flags, should be informed of their risk and provided appropriate measures to manage and prevent future breast cancer risk. Empiric breast cancer risk models can be used as a means to establish a quantitative measure of risk that can be used to implement measures to prevent or reduce breast cancer risks depending upon age, personal/family history, or other factors associated with the model (ACS, 2015; see Table 11.4). Based on empiric risk assessment, moderate risk breast cancer with a noninherited genetic mutation may still warrant enhanced surveillance (e.g., magnetic resonance imaging [MRI]), consideration of chemoprevention, and/or other therapeutic alternatives. Chemoprevention using receptor modulators (e.g., tamoxifen and raloxifene) or aromatase inhibitors (e.g., anastrozole and exemestane) may be considered to reduce breast cancer risks. For example, a woman with a 5-year Gail model risk of greater than or equal to 1.67% may be a candidate for chemoprevention to reduce her breast cancer risk and appropriate counseling should be provided to "inform" her of the advantages/disadvantages of chemoprevention (Pruthi, Heisey, & Bevers, 2015). Enhanced surveillance using MRI in addition to mammography may also be warranted for individuals based upon empiric family risk models (e.g., Claus model) that reveal a greater than or equal to 20% lifetime breast cancer risk.

TABLE 11.4 Risk Assessment (Empiric) Models for Assessment of Risk Based on Selected Personal and Family History Risk Factors

Empiric Breast Cancer Risk Assessment Model	Description
• Modified Gail model[a]— National Surgical Adjuvant Breast and Bowel Project (NSABP) P1 Study (breast cancer risk assessment tool); www.cancer.gov/bcrisktool	Empiric breast cancer risk assessment model for individuals of age 35 years and older and without a personal history of breast cancer, medical history of ductal carcinoma-in-situ (DCIS), radiation therapy to the chest for Hodgkin's lymphoma, or whose history may be suspect for a germline mutation; provides a *5-year and lifetime breast cancer risk*; assess risk based upon: (a) age; (b) age at start of menstruation; (c) age at first live birth; (d) number of first-degree relatives with breast cancer; (e) number of previous breast biopsies; (f) history of atypical hyperplasia of the breast. *Five-year risk of greater than or equal to 1.67% can be used for chemoprevention counseling to reduce risk.*
• Tyrer-Cuzick[b,c]— International Breast Intervention Study Risk Tool (IBIS); www.ems-trials.org/riskevaluator	Breast cancer risk assessment tool determines *10-year and lifetime likelihood of developing breast cancer*; incorporates: (a) family history and personal history (b) hormonal and reproductive factors; (c) age; (d) body mass index; and (e) benign breast disease.
• Claus model[d,e]—based upon data from Cancer and Steroid Hormone Study (CASH); CaGene provides a display of Claus model; www4.utsouthwestern.edu/breasthealth/cagene/default.asp	Lifetime breast cancer risk focusing on family history; considers number and ages of breast cancer in first- and second-degree relatives on maternal and paternal lineages. *Greater than or equal to 20% estimates can be used for high-risk surveillance for MRI.*

Sources: [a]NCI (2011); [b]Quante, Whittemore, Shriver, Strauch, and Terry (2012); [c]Tyrer, Duffy, and Cuzick (2004); [d]Jacobi, de Bock, Siegerink, and van Asperen (2009); [e]Bondy and Newman (2003).

Info Box

When in doubt regarding breast cancer risk, refer for evaluation of genetics (e.g., genetic counselor, advanced genetics nurse (AGN), or geneticist) to assess if genetic counseling/testing is appropriate; and refer for evaluation to a breast cancer expert (e.g., high-risk clinic) if specialized management of care is needed for individuals whose history could be suggestive of high risk.

Those individuals *suspect* for an inherited breast cancer syndrome based upon personal and/or family history should be referred for further evaluation so that genetic counseling and discussion of genetic testing, if appropriate, is provided. Genetic counseling and genetic testing (if conducted) aids in determining if a germline mutation is present that puts the individual at high breast cancer risk. Individuals with a known genetic breast cancer mutation (e.g., *BRCA; PTEN; P53*) or family history with a known genetic mutation in a patient not tested is considered high risk for breast cancer, as well as having the potential risk for other cancers or medical conditions based upon the mutation. These patients should be followed by experts in the management of high-risk breast cancer. Other risk factors like radiation exposure (e.g., radiation to the chest/mantel) may also be suggestive of high breast cancer risk depending on age and dose of exposure, requiring further management than that required for individuals considered at population or moderate breast cancer risk. Individuals at high risk for breast cancer should be informed of measures for early diagnosis or risk reduction including enhanced surveillance, chemoprevention if available, and risk-reduction surgery if applicable. Specific risk-reduction interventions are targeted to the germline mutation. For example, individuals with HBOC may consider risk-reduction surgery to reduce their breast and/or ovarian cancer risks.

Risk Counseling and Management—Genetic Testing

Identification of red flags in the personal and/or family history usually warrants further evaluation to determine if the individual should have genetic testing. Before considering genetic testing, a thorough personal and family history as well as physical examination should be conducted to determine if testing is indicated, the appropriate individual to test based upon history data, and most importantly the appropriate genetic test for consideration, if applicable. Cultural and psychosocial factors should also be a part of pre- and posttest counseling. Pretest counseling and informed consent are essential components of genetic testing. Genetic testing can be focused on assessment of gene(s) associated with a syndrome (*comprehensive analysis* [e.g. *BRCA1/2* testing for HBOC]); evaluation of a single gene based upon a known mutation in the family (*single-site mutation-specific analysis*); or founder mutations (*multisite analysis* [e.g. three-site mutation panel for Ashkenazi Jewish ancestry and HBOC: *BRCA1* 185delAG and 5382insC; and *BRCA2* 6174delT]). Often a three-site mutation panel is conducted on Ashkenazi Jewish as an initial assessment for an inherited breast cancer syndrome, particularly when HBOC is suspected as the genes analyzed in the three-site panel account for 99% of identified mutations among individuals of Ashkenazi Jewish ancestry. Multigene assessment is performed through panels. *Next-generation sequencing (NGS)* is another means of assessing for a wide range of hereditary breast cancer syndromes.

NGS incorporates multigene testing panels and is used when the personal or family history is suspect for a germline mutation and a need to assess a variety of inherited breast cancer syndromes is warranted beyond HBOC or germline *BRCA* mutations. There are a number of laboratories that conduct NGS and the type and number of genes in a panel can vary, with some panels sequencing few genes (e.g., six to eight panel: *ATM, BRCA1, BRCA2, CDH1, CHEK2, PALB2, PTEN,* and *TP53*) and other panels sequencing a far greater number of genes (e.g., 17-NGS panel (e.g., *ATM, BARD1, BRCA1, BRCA2, BRIP1, CDH1, CHEK2, MRE11A, MUTYH, NBN, NF1, PALB2, PTEN, RAD50, RAD51C, RAD51D, TP53*) and some laboratories even reporting a higher number of genes sequenced. The advantages of multigene panel testing include the number of tests and decreased costs of testing compared to testing for a single specific gene. However, this means of testing can become complex because some of the genes offered in the panels do not have a clear risk-reduction strategy (Society of Gynecologic Oncology [SGO], 2014). Further, there is an increased likelihood of identifying a variant of uncertain significance (VUS), and/or incidental findings that were not expected, and/or identification of pathogenic variants where treatment guidelines are not available or well established with NGS testing (Clifford, Hughes, Roberts,

Pirzadeh-Miller, & McLaughlin, 2016). The more the number of genes tested, the greater the likelihood of obtaining uncertain findings. Therefore, the use of multigene panel testing should be left to those with expertise (e.g., geneticist, oncologist, AGN, genetic counselor) in genetic testing, results interpretation, and risk management.

Posttest counseling of genetic testing results is an important part of genetic counseling and future risk management. The clinician should be knowledgeable of genetic results so that appropriate interpretation and communication of findings are provided to the patient. Of importance are ethical considerations of doing no harm. Noninformative test results (individuals suspect for an inherited breast cancer syndrome but results revealed no mutation) should be thoroughly assessed based on the personal and family history and appropriate risk assessment, including follow-up management of care provided as part of posttest counseling. Posttest counseling should also include discussion of cancer risk and management of care, including referral based upon the germline mutation. The Health Insurance Portability and Accountability Act (HIPAA) is also important regarding genetic test results, as notification of family members is the duty of the patient (proband/consultand) tested unless consent is obtained from the patient otherwise. A discussion with the patient regarding the genetic test results and their implication to family members is important as the patient's finding of a deleterious gene mutation usually warrants testing on other family members. In addition, a patient with a suspicious family history of breast cancer who tested "no mutation found" still may warrant other family members to consider genetic counseling and consideration of genetic testing. For example, a consultand who presents with a family history of a mother who died of breast and ovarian cancer and who obtained genetic testing where no mutation is found may still warrant her siblings or other family members to seek genetic testing to ensure that they do not have a germline mutation that the consultand did not inherit.

Ethical, legal, and social implications (ELSI) are an integral part of genetic testing and APRNs should be knowledgeable about the myriad of issues involved in this process; if not trained or experienced in cancer genetics, they should refer patients for genetic counseling to a genetic counselor, medical geneticist, or AGN with expertise and experience in cancer genetics. Chapter 8 provides additional information on risk communication and risk management including information on the genetic information and nondiscrimination act (GINA).

Hereditary Colon Cancer Syndromes

Colorectal cancer is the third most common cancer diagnosed in both men and women in the United States. The estimated lifetime risk for developing the disease for both men and women is approximately 5.0% (ACS, 2017c). Most colon cancers are sporadic (75%–80%) due to a combination of genetic and environmental factors; approximately 15% to 20% of the diseases are familial and only 3% to 5% are due to a germline mutation (Burt, 2007; NCI, 2017a). Like that of hereditary breast cancer syndromes, there are a number of hereditary CRC syndromes associated with different genes and clinical characteristics/phenotypes (Table 11.5). The *most common hereditary CRC syndrome* is Lynch syndrome (hereditary non-polyposis CRC). Of the hereditary CRC syndromes, Lynch syndrome comprises most (approximately 2% to 5%) of the individuals with a CRC germline mutation (Jasperson, Tuohy, Neklason, & Burt, 2010; NCI, 2017a). Lynch syndrome has a spectrum of conditions including colon and extra-colonic cancers, medical conditions, and skin manifestations (Table 11.5). The syndrome is due primarily to mutations in mismatch repair genes; however, a mutation in the epithelial cell adhesion molecule gene (*EPCAM*) is also associated with Lynch syndrome (da Silva, Wernhoff, Dominguez-Barrera, & Dominguez-Valentin, 2016). There are myriad cancers associated with the highly penetrant genes of Lynch syndrome; however, colon cancer (52%–82%) followed by endometrial cancer (25%–60%) and ovarian cancer (4%–24%) are the three cancers with the highest rates of cancer occurrence particularly when the germline mutation is that of *MLH1* or *MSH2* (NCCN, 2016b). *Early age onset and multiple family members* are significant in the personal and/or family history of individuals with an inherited CRC syndrome like Lynch syndrome. For example, the average age of onset for colon cancer in Lynch syndrome for most germline mutations associated with the disorder is 44 to 61 years, earlier than that of sporadic CRC (mean age ≥50); and the average age of endometrial cancer in women with a germline mutation for Lynch syndrome is 48 to 62 years (NCCN, 2016b), an age much younger than the average age of women with sporadic disease (age ≥60 years; ACS, 2017d).

Assessment is important in determining an individual's colon cancer disease risks including Lynch syndrome, and to evaluate for red flags that may be suspect for an inherited condition. The acronym RISK can be used

TABLE 11.5 Selected Inherited Syndromes Associated With Colon Cancer, and the Gene Mutation and Conditions and Cancers Associated With the Syndrome

Cancer Syndrome and (Inheritance Pattern)	Gene Mutation	Colon Cancer Risk and Risk Percentage (%), and Other Conditions Associated With the Syndrome
Lynch syndrome (AD)[a–d]	*MLH1* *MSH2* *MSH6* *PMS2* *EPCAM*	Colon cancer (52%–82%); cancers: ovarian cancer; endometrial; stomach; urinary (renal pelvis); brain (Turcot syndrome); pancreas; hepatobiliary; sebaceous neoplasma (Muir-Torre syndrome); hallmark = associated with colon, endometrial tumors—*microsatellite instability-high (MSI-H); immunohistochemical (IHC) staining absent for specific gene associated with mutation; tumor characteristics pathology—mucinous and medullary histology, signet-ring cell differentiation, and marked antitumoral immune* response[b] that often warrants further evaluation for Lynch syndrome
Familial adenomatous polyposis (FAP)[a,c,e] (AD) and *de novo* Attenuated FAP (AFAP)	*APC*	Colon cancer (~100% lifetime); ≥100 adenomatous polyps; cancer risks: medulloblastoma; papillary thyroid cancer; pancreatic; duodenal; hepatoblastoma children age younger than or equal to 5 years; extracolonic tumors: desmoid tumors; gastric fundic gland polyps
Peutz–Jeghers[c] (AD)	*STK11*	Colon cancer (39%); cancers: breast, ovarian, colorectal, gastric, pancreatic; adenoma malignum of the cervix; benign neoplasm of ovary; Peutz–Jeghers type —hamartomatous polyps: small intestine; stomach; large bowel; mucotaneous macules predominantly in childhood

(continued)

TABLE 11.5 Selected Inherited Syndromes Associated With Colon Cancer, and the Gene Mutation and Conditions and Cancers Associated With the Syndrome *(continued)*

Cancer Syndrome and (Inheritance Pattern)	Gene Mutation	Colon Cancer Risk and Risk Percentage (%), and Other Conditions Associated With the Syndrome
Cowden syndrome (AD)[c]	*PTEN*	Colon cancer (16%); cancers: breast; endometrial
MYH-associated polyposis (AR)[c,e]	*MYH*	Colon cancer (43%–53%); duodenal cancer; duodenal polyps; colon polyps usual range 0–100s; thyroid abnormalities (e.g., goiter; nodules; papillary cancer have been reported)[e]
Juvenile polyposis syndrome (AD)[c,e]	*BMPR1A* *SMAD4*	Colon cancer (40%–50%); juvenile colon polyps; gastrointestinal juvenile polyps; hereditary hemorrhagic telangiectasia risk

AD, autosomal dominant; AR, autosomal recessive.

Sources: [a]Lynch and de la Chapelle (2003); [b]Setaffy and Langner (2015); [c]NCCN (2016b); [d]da Silva et al. (2016); [e]Jasperson et al. (2010).

as a means to assess for colon cancer risk. APRNs, particularly nurse practitioners (NPs), via a comprehensive personal and family history may be the first clinician who may observe a history that may be suspect for inherited CRC syndromes; thus, the need to implement a genomic risk assessment for this condition is important.

Review of History

Personal history should include cancer history, if applicable, with age of onset, type(s) of cancer (document pathology reports, if available), treatment(s), and history of multiple primaries, if applicable. An in-depth medical history and surgical history should be included in the history assessment. Gynecological surgery performed previously should entail documentation of hysterectomy and/or oophorectomy, if applicable, including pathology findings as some inherited colon cancer syndromes are associated with endometrial and ovarian cancer like Lynch syndrome. Colon cancer screening history should consist of dates conducted and age at time of screening, type of screening (e.g., sigmoidoscopy vs. colonoscopy), presence/absence of polyps, and pathology findings of the polyps that include location, type, and number of polyps. The personal medical history is also important as a history of certain disorders (e.g., inflammatory bowel disease, ulcerative colitis, Crohn's disease) increases the risk for colon cancer (Table 11.6).

A focused exam should be conducted as part of the genomic risk assessment when evaluating individuals for an inherited CRC syndrome. The exam should focus on specific characteristics or conditions related to the syndrome. The exam might include skin, abdominal, eye, and oral examinations. For example, certain skin changes are associated with a specific form of Lynch syndrome known as Muir–Torre syndrome (e.g., sebaceous adenoma, sebaceous epithelioma, sebaceous carcinoma, keratoacanthoma). Examination of the head circumference is important as Cowden syndrome

TABLE 11.6 Factors Associated With Increasing the Risk for Colon Cancer Including Factors That May Contribute to Colon Cancer

- Prior colon cancer
- Personal history of colon polyps
- Personal history of inflammatory bowel disease
  - Personal history of ulcerative colitis
  - Personal history of Crohn's disease
- Positive family history
- Hereditary colon cancer syndromes
- Age, particularly older than 50 years
- Physical inactivity
- Nutrition history low in fruit and vegetables
- Low-fiber and high-fat diet
- Overweight/obesity
- Alcohol consumption
- Tobacco use

Sources: ACS (2017b); Centers for Disease Control and Prevention (2016); Colon Cancer Alliance (2016); NCI (2014b); NCCN (2017a).

is associated with macrocephaly and skin changes like those that occur with multiple trichilemmomas and/or papillomatous papules, particularly on the face and/or tongue (Patil et al., 2013). Eye changes with findings of a congenital hypertrophy of the retinal pigment epithelium (CHRPE; Nusliha, Dalpatadu, Amarasinghe, Chandrasinghe, & Deen, 2014), osteomas on dental examination, and/or desmoids are often found in individuals with familial adenomatous polyposis (FAP) syndrome (Groen et al., 2008; see Figures 6.1 and 6.2).

Family history should be complete and consist of preferably a three-generation history using a pedigree, if possible, on both the maternal and paternal lineages. Ancestry of origin for both lineages should be included, as well as a notation of any history of consanguinity. Cancer history data on affected relatives should be documented including current age, type of cancer, and age at diagnosis, as well as treatment(s), if known, and history of multiple primaries. Family medical history of any significant conditions should be included, particularly if the disorders are associated with specific inherited syndromes.

Identify Red Flags

Identify any potential red flags that may indicate potential genetic risk for a hereditary colon cancer syndrome (see Table 11.7).

Select a Risk Probability

The personal and family history is key to determining potential risk. If there are red flags that suggest an inherited syndrome, recommend referral consultation for further assessment and consideration for genetic counseling and possible genetic testing.

Keep Individuals Informed

Individuals without personal or familial risks are at *average/population risk* (approximately 5.0%) for colon cancer and should be informed of routine colon cancer screening based upon age. A CRC risk assessment is available to determine the risk for individuals age 50 to 85 years and whose race/ethnicity is White, African American, Hispanic/Latino, Asian, or American/Pacific Islander based upon prior studies and certain risk factors. However, the tool should *not* be used for individuals who are at increased or high risk for the disease, including those with personal history of colon cancer,

TABLE 11.7 Red Flags That Indicate Potential Risk for Inherited Colon Cancer

- Known genetic mutation in the family for an inherited colon cancer syndrome
- Early age onset colon cancer younger than age 50 or age 60 and MSI-H histology
- Multiple polyps or polyposis (e.g., FAP/AFAP; *MUTYH*-associated polyposis [MAP-1])
- Multiple family members with colon cancer on the same lineage
- Multiple family members with colon cancer and/or other cancers or conditions suggestive of an inherited colon cancer syndrome
- Endometrial cancer younger than age 50 (e.g., Lynch syndrome)
- Presence of synchronous or metachronous colorectal cancer
- Colon or endometrial cancer tumors with characteristics suggestive of Lynch syndrome (MSI-H histology; and/or IHC positive for mismatch repair gene mutation)
- Polyps suggestive of an inherited syndrome (e.g., juvenile; hamartomatous polyps)

AFAP, attenuated FAP; FAP, familial adenomatous polyposis; IHC, immunohistochemistry; MSI-H, microsatellite instability-high; *MUTYH*, (MutY Homolog of E. coli) gene that encodes an enzyme involved in DNA repair.
Sources: Jasperson et al. (2010); NCCN (2016b); NCI (2017a).

ulcerative colitis, Crohn's disease, or a hereditary colon cancer syndrome (e.g., Lynch syndrome; FAP; NCI, 2014b). The tool is available via the NCI at www.cancer.gov/colorectalcancerrisk. Colon cancer preventative measures should be discussed based on risk including lifestyle factors with proper diet, exercise, maintenance of healthy weight, and consideration of chemoprevention (e.g., aspirin) as primary preventive measures to reduce future colon cancer risks.

Individuals who are at increased risk for colon cancer based upon personal history (e.g., ulcerative colitis) or family history and whose comprehensive history is *not* suggestive of an inherited syndrome should have appropriate colon cancer screening based upon current professional guidelines and history data (e.g., NCCN guidelines).

Individuals with a diagnosed germline mutation (e.g., Lynch syndrome) are considered *high risk* and should have appropriate risk management by experts in hereditary colon cancer syndromes. Management of care for high-risk individuals is based upon the genetic mutation and diagnosis of the colon cancer syndrome. Risk management may warrant not only enhanced colon surveillance but other enhanced surveillance measures due to additional cancer risks. Based upon the inherited syndrome, for example, some syndromes may warrant further discussion of risk-reduction surgery (e.g., hysterectomy and salpingo-oophorectomy for individuals with Lynch syndrome to reduce endometrial and ovarian cancer risks) and chemoprevention.

Risk Communication and Risk Management— Genetic Testing

Personal and/or family history suggestive of an inherited colon cancer syndrome warrants genetic counseling and possible genetic testing. Because of the myriad of inherited colon cancer syndromes, genetic testing procedures may be complex with potential tumor testing required to assess for characters that may be suspect for Lynch syndrome prior to germline testing. For example, individuals with a history of colon or endometrial cancer may have evaluations of their tumors to assess for microsatellite instability-high (MSI-H) that results from a loss of the DNA mismatch repair activity (Boland & Goel, 2010). In addition, evaluation of the presence or absence of proteins associated with the specific gene expression via immunohistochemistry (IHC) may also be conducted on colon or endometrial tumors prior to conducting germline testing for Lynch syndrome. Tumors found to be MSI-H and/or show an absence of protein expression are *suspect but not diagnostic* for Lynch syndrome. The IHC tests performed by a pathologist on the tumor may be useful for assessing *MLH1, MSH2, MSH6,* and *PMS2* for presence or absence of their protein expression (Jasperson et al., 2010).

There are a number of genes associated with inherited colon cancer syndromes, and the decision on which syndrome to conduct genetic testing should be based upon one's familiarity and experience with inherited colon cancer syndromes. Further, NGS is also available for colon cancer syndromes and, like many panel tests, are complex and may lead to VUS, or incidental findings. Individuals who are suspect for an inherited CRC syndrome based upon the personal and family history should be *referred* by the APRN to a genetic counselor, medical geneticist, or AGN experienced in cancer genetics for counseling, further evaluation, and consideration for genetic testing, if appropriate.

There are a number of hereditary colon cancer syndromes, each associated with its specific germline mutation and clinical characteristics. It is important that APRNs keep abreast of hereditary cancer syndromes including those associated with CRC so that appropriate recognition and referral management can be implemented for early recognition of the syndrome through appropriate genetic testing if indicated after pretest counseling and informed consent is provided. Table 11.8 provides examples of online resources to enhance learning regarding hereditary cancer syndromes.

TABLE 11.8 Selected Online Resources on Colon Cancer and Hereditary Colon Cancer Syndromes

Online Resource	Description	Weblink
American Cancer Society	Colorectal Cancer Facts & Figures 2017–2019	www.cancer.org/content/dam/cancer-org/research/cancer-facts-and-statistics/colorectal-cancer-facts-and-figures/colorectal-cancer-facts-and-figures-2017–2019.pdf
National Cancer Institute (NCI) • Genetics of Colorectal Cancer (PDQ®)—Health Professional Version	Genetics of colorectal cancer (CRC) to include natural history of CRC; molecular events associated with colon carcinogenesis; family history as a risk factor for CRC; inheritance of CRC predisposition; and difficulties in identifying a family history of CRC risk	www.cancer.gov/types/colorectal/hp/colorectal-genetics-pdq
The Jackson Laboratory • Hereditary Colorectal Cancer Resources	Hereditary CRC resources that include tools for risk, screening, testing, ethical, legal and social issues, and risk assessment	www.jax.org/education-and-learning/clinical-and-continuing-education/colorectal-cancer-resources

(*continued*)

TABLE 11.8 Selected Online Resources on Colon Cancer and Hereditary Colon Cancer Syndromes (*continued*)

Online Resource	Description	Weblink
National Comprehensive Cancer Network (NCCN) • Genetic/Familial High-Risk Assessment: Colorectal Cancer	Clinical guidelines on selected hereditary colon cancers	www.nccn.org

TABLE 11.9 Selected Online Resources on Cancer Genetics for Clinical Practice

Online Resource	Description	Weblink
Society of Gynecologic Oncology—2016 Genetics Toolkit	Collaborative work by the Society of Gynecologic Oncology, the American College of Obstetricians and Gynecologists, the National Society of Genetic Counselors, Bright Pink, and Facing Our Risk of Cancer Empowered (FORCE): Toolkit designed to provide critical, practical information to health care providers interested in gaining understanding of the role of genetics in gynecologic cancers	www.sgo.org/genetics/genetics-toolkit
Cancer Genetics Overview (PDQ)—Health Professional Version	National Cancer Institute website that provides a wide range of information on cancer including genetics of cancer; genetics services; genetic test results; clinical DNA sequencing	www.cancer.gov/about-cancer/causes-prevention/genetics
Facing Our Risk of Cancer Empowered (FORCE)	Mission: Improve the lives of individuals and families affected by hereditary breast, ovarian, and related cancers	www.facingourrisk.org/about-us/our-impact/our-mission.php

Sources: ACS (2017a); FORCE (n.d.); The Jackson Laboratory (2017); NCI (2017a, 2017b); NCCN (2016b); Society of Gynecologic Oncology (2016).

Info Box

Approximately 2% to 5% of CRCs are due to a germline mutation (inherited). There are many hereditary CRC syndromes, each associated with a specific genetic mutation that predisposes individuals to colon cancer risks as well as extra-colonic cancers or other medical conditions. APRNs should become familiar with the syndromes so that recognition of patients with red flags suggestive of an inherited colon cancer syndrome can be referred for further evaluation, genetic counseling, and consideration for genetic testing, if indicated.

Summary

Risk assessment is an important tool to use in clinical practice to assess individuals who may be at risk for an inherited predisposition to cancer. APRNs who conduct health histories, diagnose, and treat patients (e.g., NPs, midwives) should have the knowledge and skills to recognize risk factors and red flags that may be suggestive of a hereditary cancer syndrome and provide appropriate risk communication and management to include referral when needed. Because of the continuous advances in the field of genetics, APRNs must keep abreast of issues relating to genetics/genomics including that of cancer genetics so that appropriate risk communication and management can be implemented based on an individual's probability or likelihood for disease occurrence. Table 11.9 provides additional educational resources for the APRNs pertaining to cancer genetics.

References

American Cancer Society. (n.d.). Breast cancer early detection and diagnosis. Retrieved from https://www.cancer.org/cancer/breast-cancer/screening-tests-and-early-detection.html

American Cancer Society. (2016). Breast cancer risk factors that you cannot change. Retrieved from https://www.cancer.org/cancer/breast-cancer/risk-and-prevention/breast-cancer-risk-factors-you-cannot-change.html

American Cancer Society. (2017). Probability of occurrence, dying and survival. Retrieved from http://cancerstatisticscenter.cancer.org

American Cancer Society. (2017a). *Colorectal cancer: Facts & figures 2017–2019*. Retrieved from https://www.cancer.org/content/dam/cancer-org/research/cancer-facts-and-statistics/colorectal-cancer-facts-and-figures/colorectal-cancer-facts-and-figures-2017-2019.pdf

American Cancer Society. (2017b). Colorectal cancer risk factors. Retrieved from https://www.cancer.org/cancer/colon-rectal-cancer/causes-risks-prevention/risk-factors.html

American Cancer Society. (2017c). Key statistics for colorectal cancer. Retrieved from https://www.cancer.org/cancer/colon-rectal-cancer/about/key-statistics.html

American Cancer Society. (2017d). Key statistics for endometrial cancer. Retrieved from https://www.cancer.org/cancer/endometrial-cancer/about/key-statistics.html

American Cancer Society. (2017e). What are the key statistics about breast cancer in men? Retrieved from https://www.cancer.org/cancer/breast-cancer-in-men/about/key-statistics.html

Antoniou, A. C., Casadei, S., Heikkinen, T., Barrowdale, D., Pylkas, K., Roberts, J., . . . Tischkowitz, M. (2014). Breast-cancer risk in families with mutations in *PALB2*. *New England Journal of Medicine*, *371*, 497–506.

Boland, C. R., & Goel, A. (2010). Microsatellite instability in colorectal cancer. *Gastroenterology*, *138*(6), 2073–2087. doi:10.1053/j.gastro.2009.12.064

Bondy, M. L., & Newman, L. A. (2003). Breast cancer risk assessment models. *Cancer Supplement*, *97*(1), 230–235. doi:10.1002/cncr.11018/pdf

Burt, R. (2007). Inheritance of colorectal cancer. *Drug Discovery Today: Disease Mechanisms*, *4*(4), 293–300.

Centers for Disease Control and Prevention. (2016, April 25). What are the risk factors for colorectal cancer? Retrieved from https://www.cdc.gov/cancer/colorectal/basic_info/risk_factors.htm

Clifford, E., Hughes, K. S., Roberts, M., Pirzadeh-Miller, S., & McLaughlin, S. A. (2016). Assessing, counseling, and treating patients at high risk for breast cancer. *Annals of Surgical Oncology*, *23*(1), 3128–3132.

Colon Cancer Alliance. (2016). Colon cancer risk factors. Retrieved from http://www.ccalliance.org/get-information/what-is-colon-cancer/risk-factors

Cybulski, C., Wokolorczyk, D., Jakubowska, A., Huzarski, T., Byrski, T., Gronwald, J., . . . Lubiński, J. (2011). Risk of breast cancer in women with a *CHEK2* mutation with and without a family history of breast cancer. *Journal of Clinical Oncology*, *29*(28), 3747–4752.

da Silva, F. C., Wernhoff, P., Dominguez-Barrera, C., & Dominguez-Valentin, M. (2016). Update on hereditary colorectal cancer. *Anticancer Research*, *36*(9), 4399–4405.

Eng, C. (2016, June 2). *PTEN* hamartoma tumor syndrome. In R. A. Pagon, M. P. Adam, H. H. Ardinger, S. E. Wallace, A. Amemiya, L. J. H. Bean, . . . K. Stephens (Eds.), *GeneReviews®* [Internet]. Seattle: University of Washington. Retrieved from http://www.ncbi.nlm.nih.gov/books/NBK1488

Facing Our Risk of Cancer Empowered. (n.d.). Home page—FORCE mission. Retrieved from http://www.facingourrisk.org/index.php

Ford, D., Easton, D. F., Stratton, M., Narod, S., Goldgar, D., Devilee, P., . . . Zelada-Hedman, M. (1998). Genetic heterogeneity and penetrance analysis of the *BRCA1* and *BRCA2* genes in breast cancer families. The Breast Cancer Linkage Consortium. *American Journal of Human Genetics, 62*(3), 676–689.

Groen, E. J., Roos, A., Muntinghe, F. L., Enting, R. H., de Vries, J., Kleibeuker, J. H., . . . van Beek, A. P. (2008). Extra-intestinal manifestations of familial adenomatous polyposis. *Annals of Surgical Oncology, 15*(9), 2439–2450.

Hartge, P., Struewing, J. P., Wacholder, S., Brody, L. C., & Tucker, M. A. (1999). The prevalence of common *BRCA1* and *BRCA2* mutations among Ashkenazi Jews. *American Journal of Human Genetics, 64*(4), 963–970.

Hartman, L. C., Degnim, A. C., Santen, R. J., Dupont, W. D., & Ghosh, K. (2015). Atypical hyperplasia of the breast-risk assessment and management options. *New England Journal of Medicine, 372*, 78–89.

The Jackson Laboratory. (2017). Colorectal cancer resources. Retrieved from https://www.jax .org/education-and-learning/clinical-and-continuing-education/colorectal-cancer-resources

Jacobi, C. E., de Bock, G. H., Siegerink, B., & van Asperen, C. J. (2009). Differences and similarities in breast cancer risk assessment models in clinical practice: Which model to choose? *Breast Cancer Research & Treatment, 115*(2), 381–390.

Jasperson, K. W., Tuohy, T. M., Neklason, D. W., & Burt, R. W. (2010). Hereditary and familial colon cancer. *Gastroenterology, 138*(6), 2044–2058.

Kaurah, P., & Huntsman, D. G. (2002 [Updated 2014, July 31]). Hereditary diffuse gastric cancer. In R. A. Pagon, M. P. Adam, H. H. Ardinger, S. E. Wallace, A. Amemiya, L. J. H. Bean, . . . K. Stephens (Eds.), *GeneReviews®* [Internet]. Seattle: University of Washington. Retrieved from http://www.ncbi.nlm.nih.gov/books/NBK1139

Kleibl, Z., & Kristensen, V. N. (2016, August). Women at high risk of breast cancer: Molecular characteristics, clinical presentation and management. *Breast, 28*, 136–144. doi:10.1016/breast .2016.05.006

Lee, A. J., Cunningham, A. P., Tischkowitz, M., Simard, J., Pharoah, P. D., Easton, D. F., & Antoniou, A. C. (2016). Incorporating truncating variants in *PALB2, CHEK2*, and *ATM* into the BOADICEA breast cancer risk model. *Genetics in Medicine, 18*(12), 1190–1198.

Lynch, H. T., & de la Chapelle, A. (2003). Hereditary colorectal cancer. *New England Journal of Medicine, 348*, 919–932.

Lynch, H. T., Silva, E., Snyder, C., & Lynch, J. F. (2007). Hereditary breast cancer: Part I. Diagnosing hereditary breast cancer syndromes. *Breast Journal, 14*(1), 3–13.

Mahdi, K. M., Nassin, M. R., & Nasin, K. (2013). Hereditary genes and SNPs associated with breast cancer. *Asian Pacific Journal of Cancer Prevention, 14*(6), 3403–3409.

Mai, P. L., Best, A. F., Peters, J. A., DeCastro, R. M., Khincha, P. P., Loud, J. T., . . . Savage, S. A. (2016). Risks of first and subsequent cancers among *TP53* mutation carriers in the National Cancer Institute Li-Fraumeni syndrome cohort. *Cancer, 122*(23), 3673–3681. doi:10.1002/ cncr.30248

McGarrity, T. J., Amos, C. I., & Baker, M. J. (2001 [Updated 2016, July 14]). Peutz-Jeghers syndrome. In R. A. Pagon, M. P. Adam, H. H. Ardinger, S. E. Wallace, A. Amemiya, L. J. H. Bean, . . . K. Stephens (Eds.), *GeneReviews*® [Internet]. Seattle: University of Washington. Retrieved from http://www.ncbi.nlm.nih.gov/books/NBK1266

Moskowitz, C. S., Chou, J. F., Wolden, S. L., Bernstein, J. L., Malhotra, J., Novetsky Friedman D., . . . Oeffinger, K. C. (2014). Breast cancer after chest radiation therapy for childhood cancer. *Journal of Clinical Oncology, 34*(9), 910–918.

National Cancer Institute. (2011, May 16). Breast cancer risk assessment tool. Retrieved from https://www.cancer.gov/bcrisktool

National Cancer Institute. (2014a, February 19). NIH study confirms risk factors for male breast cancer. Retrieved from https://www.cancer.gov/news-events/press-releases/2014/ BreastCancerMalePoolingStudy

National Cancer Institute. (2014b, November 12). Colorectal cancer risk factors. Retrieved from https://www.cancer.gov/colorectalcancerrisk/colorectal-cancer-risk.aspx

National Cancer Institute. (2015, April 22). The genetics of cancer. Retrieved from https://www .cancer.gov/about-cancer/causes-prevention/genetics

National Cancer Institute. (2017a, March 30 [updated]). Genetics of colorectal cancer (PDQ®)—Health professional version. Retrieved from https://www.cancer.gov/types/colorectal/ hp/colorectal-genetics-pdq

National Cancer Institute. (2017b, July 6 [updated]). Cancer genetics overview (PDQ®)— Health professional version. Retrieved from https://www.cancer.gov/about-cancer/causes -prevention/genetics/overview-pdq

National Cancer Institute. (2017c, July 13 [updated]). Genetics of breast and gynecologic cancers (PDQ®)—Health professional version. Retrieved from https://www.cancer.gov/types/ breast/hp/breast-ovarian-genetics-pdq

National Comprehensive Cancer Network. (2016a, December 7). Genetic/familial high-risk assessment: Breast and ovarian, version2.2017. Retrieved from https://www.nccn.org/ professionals/physician_gls/pdf/genetics_screening.pdf

National Comprehensive Cancer Network. (2016b, December 16). Breast cancer risk reduction, version 1.2017. Retrieved from https://www.nccn.org/professionals/physician_gls/ pdf/breast_risk.pdf

National Comprehensive Cancer Network. (2017a, May 22). Colorectal cancer screening, version 1.2017. Retrieved from https://www.nccn.org/professionals/physician_gls/pdf/ colorectal_screening.pdf

National Comprehensive Cancer Network. (2017b, June 5). Genetic/familial high-risk assessment: Colorectal, version1.2017. Retrieved from https://www.nccn.org/professionals/ physician_gls/pdf/genetics_colon.pdf

Nusliha, A., Dalpatadu, U., Amarasinghe, B., Chandrasinghe, P. C., & Deen, K. I. (2014). Congenital hypertrophy of retinal pigment epithelium (CHRPE) in patients with familial adenomatous polyposis (FAP): A polyposis registry experience. *BMC Research Notes*, 7, 734. doi:10.1186/1756-0500-7-734

Patil, P. B., Sreenivasan, V., Goel, S., Nagaraju, K., Vashishth, S., Gupta, S., & Garg, K. (2013). Cowden syndrome—Clinico-radiological illustration of a rare case. *Contemporary Clinical Dentistry*, 4(1), 119–123. doi:10.4103/0976-237X.111634

Petrucelli, N., Daly, M. B., & Feldman, G. L. (1998 [Updated 2016, December 15]). *BRCA1* and *BRCA2* hereditary breast and ovarian cancer. In R. A. Pagon, M. P. Adam, H. H. Ardinger, S. E. Wallace, A. Amemiya, L. J. H. Bean, . . . K. Stephens (Eds.), *GeneReviews®* [Internet]. Seattle: University of Washington. Retrieved from http://www.ncbi.nlm.nih.gov/books/NBK1247

Pruthi, S., Heisey, R. E., & Bevers, T. B. (2015). Chemoprevention for breast cancer. *Annals of Surgical Oncology*, 22(10), 3230–3235.

Quante, A. S., Whittemore, A. S., Shriver, T., Strauch, K., & Terry, M. B. (2012). Breast cancer risk assessment across the risk continuum: Genetic and nongenetic risk factors contributing to differential model performance. *Breast Cancer Research*, 14(6), R144. doi:10.1186/bcr3352

Ramus, S. J., Song, H., Dicks, E., Tyrer, J. P., Rosenthal, A. N., Intermaggio, M. P., . . . Gayther, S. A. (2015). Germline mutations in the *BRIP1, BARD1, PALB2*, and *NBN* genes in women with ovarian cancer. *Journal of the National Cancer Institute*, 107(11). doi:10.1093/jnci/djv214

Setaffy, L., & Langner, C. (2015). Microsatellite instability in colorectal cancer: Clinicopathological significance. *Polish Journal of Pathology*, 66(3), 203–218.

Shiovitz, S., Everett, J., Huang, S. C., Orloff, M. S., Eng, C., & Gruber, S. B. (2010). Head circumference in the clinical detection of PTEN hamartoma tumor syndrome in a clinic population at high-risk of breast cancer. *Breast Cancer Research & Treatment*, 124(2), 459–465.

Siegel, R. L., Miller, K. D., Jemal, A. (2017). Cancer statistics, 2017. *CA: A Cancer Journal for Clinicians*, 67(1), 7–30. Retrieved from http://onlinelibrary.wiley.com/doi/10.3322/caac.21387/full

Society of Gynecologic Oncology. (2014). SGO clinical practice statement: Next generation cancer gene panels versus gene by gene testing. Retrieved from https://www.sgo.org/clinical-practice/guidelines/next-generation-cancer-gene-panels-versus-gene-by-gene-testing

Society of Gynecologic Oncology. (2016). Society of Gynecologic Oncology—2016 genetics toolkit. Retrieved from https://www.sgo.org/genetics/genetics-toolkit

Streuwing, J. P., Hartge, P., Wacholder, S., Baker, S. M., Berlin, M., McAdams, M., . . . Tucker, M. A. (1997). The risk of cancer associated with specific mutations of *BRCA1* and *BRCA2* among Ashkenazi Jews. *New England Journal of Medicine*, 336(20), 1401–1408.

Tyrer, J., Duffy, S. W., & Cuzick, J. (2004). A breast cancer prediction model incorporating familial and personal risk factors. *Statistics in Medicine*, 23(7), 1111–1130.

12

Summary

Risk assessment is an important part of health care that includes early identification or prevention of disease occurrence. In this book, we present risk assessment as a continuous process in assessing for genetic/genomic risks that can have a predisposition for disease. Here we use the acronym RISK to provide essential elements of the process: *review* the history, *identify* elements of risk (red flags) that may indicate disease risk warranting further assessment like genetic testing; *select* the probability of risk through identified red flags, and *keep* the patient informed through risk communication and application of interventions for risk management. The risk assessment process aids in determining who might have an above-average population risk that may warrant evaluation for genetic testing and/or implementation of management of care interventions that may reduce disease risk.

Genetic testing has evolved over the years from *single*-gene testing to multiple-gene panel testing (expanded testing or next-generation sequencing [NGS]), which is currently used in many settings. With these tests, *multiple* genes can be tested for many conditions that represent a current disease/syndrome or for prediction of future disease. However, utilization of these measures warrants knowledge and skills of testing and appropriate patient counseling to ensure that ethical, legal, and social issues are discussed and that *maleficence* and *beneficence* are part of the informed consent process when testing is considered.

Today genetic tests are available for a wide range of uses including newborn screening, as well as diagnostic, carrier, predictive, and presymptomatic testing. Genetic testing has also played a role in pharmacogenetics where targeted testing for variants may be useful in drug choice. In the future, advance technologies will continue leading to a greater understanding of the function and interaction of genes, gene mutations, and polymorphisms that impact disease risk. These technologies hopefully will bring about better interventions to prevent and cure diseases, including the development of new drugs/medications, and to guide drug choice and/or drug dosage based on the individual's genetic profile. The future of whole genome or whole exome sequencing as well as the implication of variants regarding disease risk could play a major role in how we assess and manage patients. Advanced practice registered nurses (APRNs) providing care in clinical settings must keep abreast with these changes as they impact all aspects of patients across the life span and throughout the health and illness spectrum.

Index

Made in the USA
Las Vegas, NV
07 January 2022